INNER AND OUTER SPACE

INNER
AND
OUTER
SPACE

Introduction to a Theory
of Social Psychiatry

Richard Rabkin, M.D.

W · W · NORTON & COMPANY · INC ·

New York

301.246
R116 i
1970

For Judy

There is nothing for it but to "summon help from the Witch"—the Witch Metapsychology. Without metapsychological speculation and theorizing—I had almost said "fantasy"—we shall not get a step further.

SIGMUND FREUD

Contents

11 Preface

15 Introduction: The New Science
The Problems of Radical Solutions
Historical Review of the Development of
  Psychiatry's Role
The Three Dimensions of Depth

42 Inner and Outer Space: Dynamics
Language Structure: The Mass Noun
Early Greek Thought
The Change to Modern Thought
Criticism of Inner Space
Practical Applications in Therapy
Conclusion

60 Heat, Electricity, and Love: Dynamics
Imponderables
Affect as "a Kind of Motion"
Labeling as a Social Action
How Labeling Conflicts Are Solved
Relevance to Psychotherapy
Affect as Transaction
Implications for Treatment
Discussion

76 Topography: Is the Unconscious Necessary?
The Source of Ignorance
The Argument for the Unconscious
The Argument for Fallibility
Parapraxes, Errors, and Ignorance
Relevance to Psychotherapy
The Healing Powers of Education
Discussion

91   The Shape of Time: Epigenetics

Growth, Development, and Structure
Two-Tense and Three-Tense Languages
The History of History
Four Shapes of Time
Metachronicity
Epigenetics
Relevance to Psychotherapy

113   Energy: Economics

The Embryology of Behavior
Physiology versus Ecology
Thrasymachus' Argument
Human Ecology
Relevance to Psychotherapy

131   Social Organisms, Networks, and Interfaces: Structure

Individual and Environment
Networks
Interfaces
Conclusion

158   The Healing Fictions: Pathogenesis

Bureaucratic versus Socialized Medicine
The Placebo
The Option
The Hidden Agenda of Medical Practice
The Eclipse of the Medical Option
Ecological Consciousness
The Shape of the Social Landscape
Summary

180   Open Systems: The Theory of Treatment

Insights, Candor, and Cruelty
Significant Communications and Awareness
   Contexts
Pessimism or Optimism
Knowing How and Knowing That

197   References   209   Index

Preface

A new medicine, a new disease, and a new patient all appear in this book. In briefest summary one could say that the patient, the disease, and the medicine all reside outside of the body, in outer space, if you will, in the air between people.

For example: a girl in her late twenties living alone in New York City appeared at a hospital emergency room one night slowed in mind, hardly moving, expressing the profoundest feelings of misery and talking of suicide: in short, suffering from what a competent psychiatrist, who was immediately called to see her, called a psychotic depressive reaction. At this particular hospital and at this time in the history of psychiatry the girl would have been admitted to receive electric shock treatment but for the fact that a young resident physician assigned to the emergency room from another service inadvertently performed an experiment.

The young girl was pregnant and unmarried. In all innocence the resident inquired if she had told her parents. When she answered in the negative, he went to the phone, called the parents, and had them come down immediately. When they appeared, a classic intergenerational discussion took place:

"Why didn't you tell us . . . ?"

"I can never talk to you any more . . ."

After a two-hour discussion alone with her family, the girl went to her parent's home. Appearing for check-ups later on in the psychiatric clinic, she was no longer psychotically depressed.

The treatment in this case was like the treatment of a fractured bone. The two ends of the family were put back together again, and as with bones, some natural process of healing took place.

In this inadvertent experiment the resident treated a new patient (the family) for a disease that has no name ("a fracture") with an approach that cannot be described. It is to more clearly tell this deceptively simple story, and others like it, which can be told at present only as simple anecdotes, that this book has been written.

Each chapter is an essay on one of the areas of general theory or metapsychology. As is explained further in Chapter One, all theories in psychiatry—whether psychoanalytic, organic, or social—have in common the fact that they address similar general theoretical questions. The answers vary considerably, but each theory considers models of structure, dynamics, economics, genetics, pathogenesis, and treatment. Consequently the essays in this book are devoted to the same topics which were called by Freud "metapsychology."

Obviously each area (structure, genetics, and so forth) can be and has been the subject of an entire book. This book is intended merely to serve as an introduction. Although no final and comprehensive statement can be found, a chapter can be said to have accomplished its task if the uniqueness of social psychiatric theory has been shown.

Chapters Two, Three, and Four contain material that has appeared in somewhat different form in the *American Journal of Psychiatry* under the following titles: "Inner and Outer Space"—reprinted from volume 124, pages 335–364, 1967; "Is the Unconscious Necessary?"—reprinted from volume 125, pages 313–319, 1968; "Affect As A Social Process"—reprinted from volume 125, pages 773–779, 1968. These articles are copyright 1967 (or 1968), the American Psychiatric Association, and I am grateful for permission to reprint them.

I would like to thank my wife, Dr. Judith Godwin Rabkin. She has served as my editor, and in no small measure I owe such literacy as this book contains to her. I find that she has intuitively known all along what I preach here, and it is to this that I owe my health, sanity, and happiness.

INNER AND OUTER SPACE

CHAPTER ONE

Introduction: The New Science

> Our new science must therefore be a demonstration, so to speak, of what providence has wrought in history, for it must be a history of the institutions by which . . . providence has ordered this great city of the human race.
>
> GIAMBATTISTA VICO, 1744

There is a crucial need in psychiatry to recognize the identifying characteristics of social psychiatric theory.[1] It often seems in danger either of being assimilated into psychoana-

1. The problem of terminology is a difficult one. By *psychiatry* I mean, rather loosely, treatment in the framework of the behavioral sciences regardless of the therapist's background. By *psychoanalysis* I refer to the varied body of theory and practice of treating a one-person entity by the "talking cure." By *social psychiatry* (a term of no linguistic merit, mixing as it does Greek and Latin roots), I mean the theory and treatment practices dealing with natural groups: i.e., the theory to be developed here. Each of these terms will be further defined in the following pages.

lytic theory under such rubrics as neo-Freudianism or ego psychology, or else of being dismissed as a label with "no logical meaning" applied to the "many and heterogeneous methods of practice and prevention in the area of community mental health" (1, p. 345). Yet a point of view as old as or older than psychoanalysis, having its own heritage, outlook, and intention, should be recognized as an independent entity. This book is designed to offer examples of a distinct social psychiatric *theoretical* approach to the problems of human adaptation.

The difficulties associated with establishing social psychiatry as an independent body of thinking and method are illustrated above in Vico's use of the term *new science*. First, is it a science or only a fad? Second, to the extent that it is science, is it a new discipline or merely an addition or modification that rounds out today's psychiatry? If it *is* a new science, why is it important, and what are the problems most apt to create misunderstanding and resistance to it? Is social psychiatry as profound a theory or method of treatment as psychoanalysis, as complex as neurological theory? Or is it "supportive" rather than "reconstructive," "superficial" rather than "deep"?

At the outset we are thus faced with two major tasks: to distinguish the approach of social psychiatry from that of psychoanalysis and its modifications, and to delineate the anatomy of this particular species of psychiatry in such a fashion that its uniqueness can be appreciated. It is claimed by some that we are currently experiencing a third phase or "revolution" [2] within the mental health movement, where the former predominance of psychoanalysis is being increasingly supplanted by social and community psychiatry (2). Others disagree, claiming that it is "not really a revolution, nor an innovation; but is a definitely conservative, and perhaps even reactionary movement" (4). A third group contends that there is little unique about social psychiatry besides voguish fashions in euphemisms sparked by opportunities to obtain federal grants and funds (5), and that it is simply the "latest therapeutic bandwagon" (6). It has been noted that

2. In this context, Pinel and Freud are usually considered the leaders of the two previous psychiatric revolutions (3). Of late, it must be added, some writers tend to call the introduction of chemotherapy for mental illness in the 1950's the third revolution, and community psychiatry the fourth.

successive revisions in the name of "inpatient facilities" from *insane asylum, retreat, psychopathic hospital*, and *mental hospital* to the current term of *community mental health center* are unaccompanied by any significant change *within* such institutions. The author of the preceding remark (5) proceeds to question whether there is any theory at all associated with the various terms connected with the "third revolution," which must include "social psychiatry."

This challenge to social psychiatry is an appropriate one. An incidental finding in a current study of psychiatric ideologies demonstrates the need for clarifying the role of social psychiatry as a distinct theory. Its authors found that among psychiatrists, three ideological types emerged: those who endorse psychoanalytic principles and assumptions, those with a predominantly neurological orientation, and those favoring social psychiatry. The social psychiatric group seemed generally compatible with either of the other two groups, apparently having no conflicting philosophy but simply a benevolent concern for maximizing treatment possibilities (7). In this study, the attitudes and beliefs of individual psychiatrists were polled, not the nature of their underlying theoretical assumptions. Because of the pragmatic and concrete nature of the survey items used, the investigation apparently identified all those non-neurological practitioners who have become aware, through practical necessity, of treatment methods other than psychoanalysis. It has not defined the smaller group whose work methods derive specifically from their involvement in the broader context of social psychiatric theory. The orientation of social psychiatry was *initially* adopted in many places because of prevailing contingencies rather than intellectual preference. For example, in many hospitals, especially state institutions in less populated areas, psychoanalytically or neurologically oriented psychiatrists were simply not available, and it was largely for this reason that hospital administrators became aware of the therapeutic effectiveness of other family members, other patients, nurses, and other auxilliary personnel. Even now the majority of those who might be called social psychiatrists are largely oblivious to the theoretical rationale of their method, although the growing subspeciality of family therapy includes many who do identify the intellectual origins of their approach. It is thus not surprising that at least one observer has commented on the "spectacle" of the "Babel syndrome" in which social psychiatry as a term is used by professionals without their knowing how their colleagues interpret the term (8).

There is, unfortunately, a failure among all psychiatrists to distinguish and to be concerned about underlying philosophies or "general theories." As David Rapaport has said of psychoanalytic theory, "The general [in contrast to the clinical] theory, far from being well-ingrained dogma, is a waif unknown to many, noticed by some, and closely familiar to few. Not the alleged rigidity of the theory, but rather unfamiliarity with it is the obstacle to theoretical progress" (9, p. 163). In a similar vein, a commentator remarked about neo-Freudians that "the trouble with the 'revisionists' of Freud . . . is not so much their ideas—many of which, emphasizing the social molding of human nature, are valuable. . . . It is the utter lack of any system, of intellectual coherence, of decisiveness; the neo-Freudians seem to live intellectually from hand to mouth" (10, p. 376).

In psychiatry, ideological incompatibility usually develops when the same set of assumptions is used as the basis for widely differing positions, as in the dispute between adherents of psychoanalytic and neurological points of view. For example, both of these groups accept the medical model and the notion of distinct disease entities such as schizophrenia, but disagree on their origins and preferred treatment techniques. It is seldom recognized that social psychiatry differs from the other positions in terms of its *assumptions* and therefore cannot legitimately be compared solely in terms of its conclusions. That it is a non-competitive approach is apparent only when it is recognized as a distinct body of ideas that stands by itself. If this basic distinction is *not* acknowledged, social psychiatry will be seen as belligerently disputing the accuracy of psychoanalytic or neurological deductions (mistakenly, for they are deduced by logical men), rather than peacefully exploring different fundamental assumptions.

Social psychiatric thought historically has been plagued by well-meaning efforts to integrate its tenets with the totally incompatible point of view of psychoanalysis. In many instances, schools of thought such as those of Adler or Sullivan were labeled neo-Freudian or Revisionist, although their founders objected to such efforts at assimilation. Because their work was seen as filling

in or developing areas of psychoanalytic theory rather than recognizing their philosophical independence, ideological battles developed without any real basis. It is thus imperative to distinguish
social psychiatry from psychoanalysis not only in practical terms
but on a theoretical basis as well. As developed in this book, social psychiatric theory is of no practical value to psychoanalysts or
neurologically-oriented psychiatrists except to the extent that
they are interested in a completely different field—as different as
ornithology.

It is likely that psychoanalysts have tended to encompass dissident branches of theory and treatment under their aegis both as a
sign of respect for their founders and also as a means of maintaining their status and power within American psychiatry. During
the last decade or so, as interest in treating psychiatric problems
of lower-class patients has increased, modified methods of traditional psychoanalysis have been developed. It is in this vague area
of "supportive therapy" that much of social psychiatry was placed
until it burst forth as its own master when President Kennedy
called on psychiatry for a "bold new approach" in 1963 (11).
Pressure built up to assimilate social psychiatry as a modification
of psychoanalysis, to return it to the fold, while efforts were made
to incorporate the insights of social psychiatry into that of psychoanalysis. These approaches satisfy neither conservative psychoanalysts nor independent social psychiatrists, who largely
agree that their respective theories differ in terms of basic conceptual foundations rather than details. When men disagree at this
level, ideological conflicts do not appear, and they are able to respect the ideas of the other point of view as valuable but unrelated to their own fields of study.

In short, the frequency of the more common criticisms of social
psychiatry have tended to block the practical applications of the
ideas of philosophers as well as the philosophical reflections of
psychiatric practitioners. Thus, dismissing social psychiatry by
calling it a grab-bag of new terms for old and conservative methods stifles the practical application of the works of such men as
John Dewey and Gilbert Ryle, philosophers who have written extensively about "mental life" from a point of view that is essentially social psychiatry. On the other hand, efforts to assimilate social psychiatry into psychoanalytic theory creates needless conflict

and suppresses the philosophical distinctions evolved by such men as Harry Stack Sullivan, a psychiatrist who practiced social psychiatry before the term was invented.

THE PROBLEMS OF RADICAL SOLUTIONS

When Vico in 1744 spoke of "this great city of the human race," he was, of course, speaking metaphorically. Not until today, when his metaphor approaches a reality, is the new science he espoused considered a serious need. In 1900 more than half of the American population lived on farms and most of the rest in small towns. Today something like 5 percent of our population is rural, and this proportion continues to dwindle while urban agglomerations expand. For example, in the next thirty-two years, the population of the greater New York metropolitan area is expected to increase by 58 percent to thirty million. It thus becomes ever more compelling for us to promote the development of a science designed to cope with the social problems created by this form of population distribution. It is quite apparent that any system of theory and techniques that focuses on prevention of psychiatric problems in large social groups has an immediacy and relevance that the individually oriented psychiatry of the last two hundred years does not possess (11). It is unfortunate that Vico's concern was not heeded long ago: "Whoever reflects on this cannot but marvel that philosophers should have bent all their energies to the study of the world of nature, which, since God made it, He alone knows; and that they should have neglected the study of the world of nations, or civil world, which, since men made it, men could come to know" (12, p. 53).

Since traditional psychiatry cannot either conceptually or practically cope with or even define contemporary social problems, it is not surprising that voices from a variety of sources are calling for new solutions. For example, Vico's concern with the "civil world" is echoed in recent federal legislative proposals which attempt to focus attention on social and other problems of the cities. At present, two bills of this sort are pending: one would establish a National Social Science Foundation to support research, and the other would establish a Council of Social Advisors and authorize an annual Social Report to Congress analogous to the existing economic reports that are regularly prepared. Other parallel and sometimes redundant attempts have been made to encourage "bold new approaches" (11), "maverick research" (13, p. 908), and "innovative, bold, original and controversial" (14) thinking.

Although the need is obvious, the problem can hardly be called new, since Vico commented on it and outlined a science directed at its solution in the early 1700's. Furthermore, there exists a variety of difficulties and sources of resistance associated with the kind of radical new "answers" which are now in demand and which have not been adequately investigated. Some of these are related to the historical relationships between living conditions and the explanatory systems adopted to account for men's behavior, and others concern the consequences that follow radical changes in such conceptual formulations.

Regardless of the extent to which the business of self-knowledge has been promoted as the ultimate concern of mankind, we have been extremely conservative in our thoughts about who and what we are. In fact, there appear to have been only three major shifts in thinking about ourselves in the history of Western thought. Each of these eras was characterized by a set of metaphors or models meant to account for human behavior. First there was the divine machinery of ancient Greece, according to which gods prompted and controlled men's behavior. Next came the inner machinery of the Iron Age, lasting from about 1000 B. C. to the present, where inner processes, urges, and motivations were seen as the regulating sources of behavior. The third era is the present, consisting of those new solutions proposed by a variety of thinkers in such diverse fields as British and American philosophy, general systems theory, the "new biology," and social psychiatry.

It is inaccurate to regard these periods of ideas as linear, successive, or fixed, although it is simpler to describe and discuss them as such. Many ideas percolate for a long time before rising to the surface to be acknowledged and accepted. This seems true of Vico's thinking about social organizations: similar notions are now rising everywhere like air bubbles to the surface of a pot about to boil.

Each of these eras has been distinguished by a shift in conceptual organization to a new level of generalization. This kind of shift characteristically accompanies creative problem-solving, whether the problem at hand is petty or profound. Consider the following riddle: A professor is walking on the Bowery. A bum lying drunk and dirty in a doorway says, "Hello, brother." The professor is, in fact, the alcoholic's brother, but the alcoholic is not the professor's brother. Who is the bum?

As I noted, creative problem-solving often entails a conceptual shift or change of context. This often takes the form of moving to a higher plane of generality, the formation of a superordinate concept. The simple riddle posed here seems puzzling because most of us think in terms of a frame of reference where bums are men. As soon as we think more generally about family relationships, its solution becomes obvious.

The principal discoveries of the Iron Age consisted of new conceptual tools and frames of reference not available in the earlier Bronze Age. Although the availability of iron may have been the stimulus for the start of this era, it is more properly defined by these conceptual tools. We may not recognize them because for twenty-five hundred years they have formed the very atmosphere in which we live. Instead we tend to study specific philosophies and men. From a contemporary point of view, Bronze Age man and his beliefs are usually seen as primitive in the sense of inferior. For instance, in that era there was no concept of mind. But these men were not simpletons who overlooked such "basic" assumptions as the mind out of sheer inferiority. They were sophisticated men, of the very same species as we, whose living conditions made it useless to work with or think about the notion of an individual, subcutaneous executive unit. Tribal man and detribalized man need, and therefore invent, different concepts. This raises some disturbing questions. If, as McLuhan has claimed, it is true that the ongoing population increase is such that it can no longer be thought of as an explosion but is rather an "implosion," a falling in on ourselves or a *re-tribalization* (15), are we not then in need of reinstituting Bronze Age beliefs? McLuhan has noted that : " . . . we are experiencing the same confusions and indecisions which they [the Elizabethans] had felt when living simultaneously in two contrasted forms of society and experience. Whereas the Elizabethans were poised between medieval corporate experience and modern individualism, we reverse their pattern by confronting an electronic technology which would seem to render individualism obsolete and the corporate interdependence mandatory" (15, p. 50). Is it then time to jettison our current models of ourselves and return to the extrapsychic models of early Greece, whose vestiges still remain in the backwaters of our culture in such forms as astrology and spiritualism? Is it a coincidence that hippie semitribal communes become involved in this sort of thinking, or is it a correlate of their social organization? It is suggested that such conceptual regression is not in fact necessary and that social psychiatry need not be a conservative force. At the same time it is necessary to acknowledge that we are living at the interface or meeting ground between the late Iron Age and whatever is to follow. We must consequently be prepared to see our belief systems change. It is also well worth noting that the last major change in systems of thought and social organization, between the Bronze and Iron Ages, was followed by centuries of chaos.

It is in view of such considerations that well-meaning requests for bold, new, innovative, and original approaches to the problems of our society seem to possess a double naivete in thinking, first, that maintenance of existing conditions is even feasible, and second, that radical change can be brought about smoothly. In other words, those who call for radical change are acting as if it would not otherwise materialize. They bring to mind the fable of the mouse who climbed onto the head of an elephant and imagined himself to be its driver or *mahout*. To preserve this illusion, when the elephant moved in one direction, the mouse subsequently called out the command. In short, it looks very much as though bold new social theories will appear anyway. The second point is that seekers of radical change are naive in ignoring the prolonged and utter chaos that is likely to follow the demise of the present social system.

HISTORICAL REVIEW OF THE DEVELOPMENT OF PSYCHIATRY'S ROLE

It seems generally true that one source of resistance to new theory is related to its effect on existing professions, just as one of the resistances to a new profession stems from its effect on existing theory. Since social psychiatry involves both new theory and new personnel, it becomes relevant to observe the traditional theory and professional identities that may be challenged by its appearance. The established theory of the mental health fields has already been noted; the characteristics of the professions themselves as they evolved in the twentieth century will be presented in this section. This survey has the added value of demonstrating on a smaller scale the consequences that radical conceptual and systemic change can bring about along lines observed earlier in this chapter.

There have developed in twentieth-century American psychiatry two separate and largely independent branches. One, concerning adults, is largely associated with hospitals, where treatment consisted almost exclusively of custodial care. The other, initially intended for children only, is based in outpatient clinics or child guidance centers, as they have come to be known. Since most of the talent, innovative effort, theory, and money has been devoted to the latter, it is this branch which best represents the mainstream of thought and practice in the mental health field during the past sixty years.

In the United States, psychiatric diagnosis and treatment outside of hospitals historically has been organized in terms of interdisciplinary cooperation between psychiatrists, psychologists, and social workers, who have functioned as an "orthopsychiatric team," virtually devoid of contact with other fields of medicine or social science.[3] Such teams have a hierarchical structure in terms of power, responsibility, and social and financial status, with the psychiatrist in charge, followed by psychologist and social worker in that order. These teams evolved over a period of several decades and functioned in a closed world with their own language, caste, problems, and standards.

The Chicago Juvenile Court Clinic, set up by William Healy in 1909, was the first American child guidance clinic as we now know them. The original impetus for its establishment stemmed not from psychiatric interests, but rather from those related to

3. For a recent, different, and more favorable historical interpretation than what is to follow see "Special Section, Orthopsychiatry, Its History, Its Future" in the *American Journal of Orthopsychiatry,* vol. 38 (1968), 799–813.

court reform. A reorganization in the Chicago judicial system led to the establishment of special children's courts for juvenile offenders. Soon the issue of justice, with respect to verdicts and sentences, was superseded by efforts to understand the delinquent behavior with a view toward rehabilitation and prevention on a broader scale. At this point Healy's clinic was established by the Juvenile Protective Association to work in conjunction with the juvenile court. Soon after, a small pilot project sponsored by this Association was undertaken to collect data demonstrating the utility of the court clinic. Healy, its physician-director—apparently a charismatic individual—wanted to publish his findings but the Association did not feel that his results were adequate. Healy discovered that the woman whose contributions maintained the clinic for the Association was willing to continue her support. The Juvenile Protective Association then severed its connections with the clinic, but by then it was too late. Inadequately evaluated patterns had been established which were to continue until the present, not only in court clinics but in psychiatry generally. An understanding of delinquency and a preventative social program were never actually accomplished by Healy, who subsequently became interested in psychoanalysis and another category of patients and problems (16).

When Healy first established his clinic he was faced with the unfortunate fact that there were no professionals trained for the type of work he envisaged. The prevailing orientation of psychiatry was then Kraepelinian—a name referring to a German school of descriptive psychiatry which placed almost exclusive emphasis on diagnosis on the assumption that disease outcome was a function of the specific syndrome; this allowed little room for believing in the effectiveness of therapeutic intervention. Children were regarded as miniature adults, psychiatrically speaking, and it was assumed that knowledge of adult disease entities was the only prerequisite for work with children. Psychiatric social work did not then exist, although the settlement house movement (a forerunner of group work) was actively trying to deal with the problems of poverty. American psychology was largely academic; clinical psychology as a subspecialty was not yet recognized. The psychological tests so widely used today had not been invented, and the small group of psychologists interested in clinical problems were just then becoming acquainted with the Binet intelligence test. Healy's solution was to develop a fourfold approach to the examination of children which utilized a pediatrician, psychologist, probation officer or volunteer (later a social worker), and psychiatrist. Today, the pediatrician's physical examination is left out and the remaining three workers are called the "orthopsychiatric team."

The nationwide proliferation of child guidance clinics began in the 1920's, when the mental hygiene movement through the National Committee for Mental Hygiene and the Commonwealth Fund subsidized five hundred demonstration clinics modeled after Healy's invention. Today there is hardly an American city that does not have its own guidance clinic. It is interesting to note that these clinics were originally founded for the "prevention of delinquency," but that neither prevention nor delinquency became their primary concerns. Non-legal psychiatric problems soon came to occupy the bulk of the caseloads, and juvenile delinquents received proportionately less attention. It is not clear how non-court cases came to the clinics, although referral sources were never exclusively limited to the courts. Healy himself noted that by 1947, only 10 percent of the referrals at the child guidance clinic where he then worked—Judge Baker Clinic in Boston—came from the juvenile courts (16).

In 1924 the establishment of the American Orthopsychiatric Association served to crystallize the roles and organization of the members of the three disciplines involved. The term *orthopsychiatry*, strongly endorsed by Karl Menninger, referred to "straightening out" the mind but still carried strong connotations of the correctional and judicial systems. An alternate name offered to the Association by a dissenting group was "social psychiatry." Particularly on Menninger's advice this term was rejected because it was said to obscure the distinction his faction wished to establish between sociology-anthropology and psychiatry—a problem that the term *orthopsychiatry* merely served to delay until the present.

Court reform and the initial emphasis on juvenile delinquency established the individual child as the focus of study, just as he was the focus of courtroom procedure. The psychologist tested the child, the social worker spoke to his parents about him, and the psychiatrist gave the child a mental status examination in a verbal interview. At the end of this procedure, the results were compiled and advice was given to the court about the child. As schools and parents began to replace the courts as major referral sources, they in turn were given advice and instructions about what to do with the child. In general, direct and intensive intervention was not undertaken until the 1930's, when psychotherapeutic efforts with the child were introduced under the auspices of the newly prominent psychoanalytic school of thought. The degree of naivete of the early method is illustrated by this example: "In an early case, Dr. Healy asked a child, "What do you think of just before you take something?" "I think about John. If I see it in my reading lesson, I must take something." Suddenly he had poured out an experience that had evidently been repressed below the conscious level. The stealing stopped from that moment . . ." (16).

It was the use of case illustrations as sole evidence for a rather elaborate clinic system, in place of detailed research, that led the original group of supporters to withdraw their endorsement of the child guidance establishment. Interestingly enough, it was rather similar material—follow-up studies that demonstrated the ineffectiveness of the clinics' advice—that led the clinics to abandon this approach (maintaining nevertheless that the children would have improved if their advice had been followed). Instead, a psychoanalytic orientation entailing intensive and "deep" work with the individual child over a protracted period of time was adopted. By 1938, Jenkins reports that the earlier emphasis on diagnosis had been largely replaced by concern with treatment, to the extent that diagnosis was regarded as a waste of time (17).

Psychoanalytically oriented psychotherapy dominated practices in child guidance clinics from the late 1930's, when European refugee analysts began to appear on the American scene, until the early 1960's, and in many clinics continues to prevail. The theoretical orientation of psychoanalysis influenced both the selection of patients and the nature and extent of treatment. Since its methods are predicated on the absence of ongoing environmental trauma or severe current psychopathology, and usually require a certain level of intelligence, verbal ability, and capacity for introspection and self-report, the practical though probably unintended effect was to exclude from treatment whatever proportion of lower-class families had formerly been served at such clinics. In the course of treatment, which often lasted for one to three years, the essential problems dealt with were those seen as species-wide, such as the Oedipus complex and separation anxiety. Treatment was based on the assumption that the individual is inevitably born into illness, since illness was defined as conflict between inner impulses and either ego, superego, or society at large. It was further assumed that anyone could benefit from psychoanalytic treatment if he had the basic tools with which to participate meaningfully and were not too sick. As Rieff (18) has noted, psychoanalysis is essentially a "therapy for the healthy, not a solution for the sick."

The impact of psychoanalytic theory on the orthopsychiatric team and its characteristic modes of functioning was disruptive. The team approach had been reasonably effective until then, but now was faced with a variety of problems. Psychoanalysis did not make the same status distinctions between psychiatrist, psychologist, and social worker that had prevailed earlier; a staff member was either psychoanalytically-oriented and trained or he was not. The specific skills that had earlier differentiated the various professionals—testing, social background studies, mental status examinations—were no longer relevant to the major task of the clinic, which came to be seen as treatment. One of the initial solutions was for each member of the team to see himself as treating a separate individual. The highest-ranking team member, the psychiatrist, saw the child, while psychologists and social workers saw the parents, or else the latter saw the child and the psychiatrist supervised their therapeutic efforts—itself a quasi-treatment situation. At this point it was a bewildering problem: " . . . most of us reacted to the apparent confusion by attempting to define more sharply the separate disciplinary roles and functions. . . . Various attempts were made to establish complex administrative procedures and definitions of roles which would protect the identity of the disciplines. In brief, it seemed as though we were engaged in a desperate attempt to maintain the old order and arrest the healthy flowering of the three disciplines into mutually supportive, healthy agents. . . ." (19, p. 349).

Such efforts were interspersed with those seeking the establishment of a single profession of psychotherapy where the training would not lead to the M.D. of the psychiatrist or the Ph.D. of the psychologist but to a special professional degree. Some educational leaders in the respective disciplines still continue to seek the organization of a training program of this nature.

While the orthopsychiatric team was experiencing internal difficulties through the 1940's, paradoxically created by the disruption of old status relationships which followed the spread of psychoanalytic orientation, the respective members still struggled to work out compatible roles within the system. Their troubles were subsequently compounded by the decline experienced by the psychoanalytic movement itself. By the early 1960's, both popular and professional interest in psychoanalysis began to diminish after the peak of its popularity following World War II. A variety of factors contributed to this situation. Public disenchantment with psychoanalysis is probably largely due to the disappointment of unrealistic expectations built up when the mass media first began to generate enthusiasm about this marvelous new method said to end divorce, crime, problems of childhood, and a host of other social ailments. Although the analysts themselves never promoted such utopian hopes, these expectations were fairly common until it began to be apparent that psychoanalysis was not as magical as initially believed. Other factors contributing to a decline of public enthusiasm were the enormous expense in terms of both money and time involved in psychoanalysis, coupled with the absence of satisfactory data showing the effectiveness of the method, either by itself or in comparison to quicker and less expensive therapeutic techniques.

Among professionals, disenchantment with psychoanalysis derived from such factors as organizational and instructional difficulties of the method. Psychoanalytic training facilities had relatively few openings, so that the extensive training required was not available to many. The orthodox psychoanalytic institutes in America accepted only physician candidates, excluding all other applicants. On the other hand, many analysts came to hold positions of prominence in the psychiatry departments of medical schools (about one-quarter of the department chairmen are now analysts), and taught all psychiatric residents rather diluted psychoanalytic theory, leading many young psychiatrists to feel that the arduous training of the institutes was no longer necessary, that they knew enough about psychoanalysis to consider and call themselves analysts. This diffusion weakened the psychoanalytic movement in several ways. It led to the realization of one of Freud's worst fears: that psychoanalysis would be presented as one of several alternative methods (among others are shock treatment, family therapy, chemotherapy), rather than the fundamental approach to the study of personality. Factors that detracted from the status of psychoanalysis among professional circles were the unwillingness of the orthodox American Psychoanalytic Association to move with the times, and the irrelevance of psychoanalysis as a treatment method for the very sick and the socially disadvantaged—who after all made up the bulk of those most in need of psychiatric assistance. Other critics have noted the lack of productive research, and the concern of the academic community that "this revolution, like all others, may already have become an orthodoxy" (20, p. 60). A final problem to be mentioned in this context is the change in the type of people who are psychoanalysts. The first group in the United States were predominantly European refugees who were broadly educated in the humanities, philosophically oriented, and experienced in living. Psychoanalysis for them was a way of life. Today, when fees are typically thirty-five dollars an hour, it has become more frequently a way of making a living. As Norman Mailer recently noted: "People in analysis began to be subjected to men who were no longer cultivated, poetic, deep and engaged in intellectual activity, but to men who were technicians, essentially interested in dominating the material before them, treating them as a commodity, as a machine to be successfully redesigned" (21).

In short, adoption of orthodox or modified psychoanalysis as a prevailing orientation by the child guidance clinics failed to provide them with a satisfactory means of serving the general public. It led to the disruption of the carefully worked out relationships between the professions that the clinics had more or less created: psychiatric social work, clinical psychology, and dynamic psychiatry.[4] At the same time, the psychoanalytic base was in flux and in the process of being diluted, criticized, and modified by its initial success in academic circles.

4. I have omitted any complete history of these professions. Psychiatric social work flourished after World War I within the state mental hospital system (22), while clinical psychology received its greatest impetus following World War II in the Veterans Administration hospital system. Despite these hospital contexts, the main patterns of relationships between these professions and psychiatry were established and predominantly influenced by events within the child guidance movement.

Another factor that served to detract from the position of psychoanalysis and the functioning of the orthopsychiatric team was the revitalization of a native American movement which had been dominant in nineteenth-century psychiatry but which had subsided around 1900, leaving the vacuum which Healy's clinic was established to fulfill. This movement or orientation had approached the treatment of the mentally ill from the point of view of the social sciences rather than medicine. Prior to the Civil War and the great waves of immigration at the end of the nineteenth century, American treatment of psychiatric patients in small New England hospitals had been remarkably successful. Recovery rates for patients admitted within a year of onset of their disturbance were as high as 90 percent. A hundred years later, in 1933, the overall recovery rate of hospitalized mental patients had dropped to 4 percent (23), although the proportion of hospital admissions relative to the total population remained about the same (24). The interplay of factors culminating in the horror of the twentieth-century "warehouses for the unwanted" has been summarized by Bockhoven (23):

1. The large number of men killed in the Civil War led to a radical change in employment patterns within mental hospitals, reducing the pool of available aides and attendants considerably.

2. The influx of patients from poverty-stricken immigrant families ("foreign insane pauperism") upset payment schemes, social and physical structures within hospitals ("those people don't need curtains on the window"), and thus associated psychiatric facilities with cheap, humiliating surroundings while other kinds of hospitals were becoming more popularly accepted and respected as places to go for successful treatment rather than simply for terminal cases.

3. The early leaders of the humane, psychological treatment programs did not train enough men to replace them, and as they left the scene, a vacuum was created.

4. There was a failure to plan ahead and create a sufficient number of small, community-based hospitals, with the result that severe overcrowding became a chronic problem.

5. The rise of the mental hygiene movement in the 1890's, championed by Clifford Beers and Dorothea Dix, led to a crusade for the identification of the mentally ill, their removal from jail or home, and much needed corrections of the abuses to which

they were often subjected. But by creating the need for more facilities and inundating existing ones with newly discovered
chronic patients, these well-meaning reformers finished off the
earlier treatment programs without supplying solutions for the
bureaucratic corruption and incompetence of the enormous new
mental institutions that came into being as a product of their la-
bors.

6. In addition, these reformers destroyed the theoretical base of
"moral" or social treatment and led to the introduction of an organic orientation which has been described as "regressively pre-
Pinel." This orientation attributed mental illness to physiological
deficit or impairment, which made psychological and social treatment irrelevant and logically futile.

The treatment that was so effective in the small, financially
sound, homogeneous Yankee community hospitals of the early
nineteenth century was called moral treatment. To review in brief
the evolution of moral or social psychiatry: it depended on the establishment of a therapeutic atmosphere derived from European
sources like those of Pinel and the York Retreat, whose philosophical dimensions were subsequently expanded by such Americans as Thoreau, Emerson, Dewey, and Mead. No clear description of the background of this American school is available. It is
best seen by following threads through the work of Thoreau, to
the Metaphysics Club at Harvard (Peirce and James), to the Chicago group (Dewey, who was championed by James; G. H. Mead,
who tutored James' children; Cooley; and Thomas). Following
this was a period in which various disciplines in the social sciences developed, such as sociology, anthropology, general seman-
tics, and social psychology. Treatment of mental patients, which
in the early 1800's was founded in this context, parted company
from this orientation until the late 1920's, when the psychiatrists
William Alanson White and H. S. Sullivan conducted a series of
interdisciplinary seminars with the social sciences. Working
within this context, Sullivan was able to approach the discharge
rate of the earlier treatment era by using similar principles. This
approach to psychiatry as a social science was unfortunately interrupted by World War II, after which psychoanalysis emerged as
the new frontier of psychiatric treatment and overshadowed the
less developed and cohesive group of ideas and practices known
collectively today as social psychiatry.

In recent years there has emerged a group, lacking a strong financial, organizational, or prestigious base, that has come to take exception to the theory and structure of the mental health field as it has evolved. Among social workers and psychologists, an increasing number have bemoaned the economics and status considerations which led many in their professions to emulate the psychiatrist's private practice of psychotherapy to the point of becoming second-class psychiatrists. Psychologists, for example, are beginning to criticize the postwar strategy of psychology graduate schools in using the Veterans Administration hospital system's money, medical framework, and role within the orthopsychiatric team to establish psychology training programs and internships (25). The size and impact of these dissident voices, coinciding as they did with the rise of a civil rights movement seeking adequate health and mental health care for the enormous numbers of poor who had been receiving largely custodial psychiatric care, developed sufficient strength to generate congressional interest and concern.

The Joint Commission on Mental Health and Illness was established in 1955 to carry out "an objective, thorough, nationwide analysis and re-evaluation of the human and economic problems of mental illness." The tremendous dimensions of the mental hygiene problem, the inadequate numbers of trained personnel, the limitations of the clinic setting, and the lack of preventative programs were among the major findings of the Commission, submitted in its 1961 report. These findings provided a license, an impetus, and a base for those who wished to venture in a new direction: social and community psychiatry. Its effect on the demise of the orthopsychiatric team is becoming apparent. With the emergence of social psychiatry as the major contemporary frontier of psychiatry the cycle has run full circle. Once again we are in Healy's position. There are no trained professionals with the needed skills to operate the programs envisaged by social psychiatry, and the delinquent and the poor are once again of primary concern. Most ironic, court reform—this time sought by civil rights and civil liberties groups concerned with loss of due process and liberty by involuntary commitment to mental hospitals or clinics—is again a live issue, as are adequate evaluation, research, and accountability to the community. Those invested in the traditional orthopsychiatric team are understandably opposed to or at least uninterested in this new framework; among them, psychiatrists, who have the most to lose, are apt to be most conservative.

While ferment and change occur within the mental health professions, major new developments in the social sciences may actually supersede the former in terms of ultimate social impact and change. Individual members of a great variety of academic and professional fields such as sociology, architecture, city planning, political science, economics, and biology have become interested and involved in a little-known but increasingly important task: planning the future. Their work is predicated on the assumption that, as Bell states it, "in the decisions we make now, in the way we design our environment and thus sketch the lines of constraints, the future is committed" (26, p. 639). He sees as the task of future-planners "to indicate now the future consequences of present public-policy decisions, to anticipate future problems, and to begin the design of alternative solutions so that our society has more options and can make a moral choice, rather than be constrained, as is so often the case when problems descend upon us unnoticed and demand an immediate response" (26). The proximity of the year 2000 has provided a convenient landmark of the future, and there exist several projects such as the Commission on the Year 2000, the Futurists, and the Committee on the Next Thirty Years, designed to meet such goals. These groups presently exist at the international and national levels, and hundreds of large corporations and foundations have future-planning operations.

Much of this work crosses so many disciplinary and professional lines as to constitute a type of superordinate academic force which reorganizes and formulates material so that it seems derived not specifically from any given profession, but rather from "social science" in general. The future-planners are said to dream, for example, of "using social science instead of pressure politics to solve the nation's problems" (27, p. 1037). In practice, however, many of the methods and approaches thus prescribed are equivalent to those of psychiatry, applied to the community rather than the individual. If the task of psychotherapy is conceptualized as changing the behavior of the patient along lines that are mutually acceptable to patient and therapist, then the task of future-planning may be considered as involving psychotherapeutic treatment of the community as a whole. There is one basic difference: while almost all patients themselves voluntarily initiate treatment, members of communities have not themselves sought such services directly. The overlapping characteristics of future-planning and psychiatry become more apparent when we think about current mental health practices and intentions.

In 1963, federal legislation authorized the establishment of mental health centers throughout the entire country, organized to serve specific districts or "catchment areas." These centers are in fact generally sponsored or set up by existing hospitals, which are assigned responsibility for the mental health of the area's inhabitants. This raises a variety of legal and ethical problems regarding the extent to which governmental intervention is justified, issues of individual privacy and independence. It is not unrealistic to contemplate a situation in which those who are disturbing the existing social order are seen as needing the psychiatric attention of the local mental health center which has the responsibility for their mental health. At some point the distinction between government intervention of this nature and the establishment of "thought police" becomes obscured.

The extent to which it is justifiable to use psychiatric techniques in the promotion of social change has long aroused controversy. A similar problem prevailed before World War II, when a segment of psychiatry then too had begun to address itself to various social problems. Lasswell wrote at the time, "By grace of his psychiatry, of course, the modern philosopher who would be king knows that he may lose his philosophy on the path to the throne, and arrive there empty of all that would distinguish him from the king whom he has overthrown" (28, p. 39). This problem of the philosopher king has been debated since Plato's time. Today it is not the philosopher but the social scientist who seems headed for the seat of power through exercise of techniques to influence the behavior of communities. The possibility that social science or psychiatry could or would replace political science or practical politics raises the specter of an efficient, psychologically oriented dictatorship—a romantic notion similar to the hopes pinned on propaganda in earlier years. Kopkind imagines a scene in the 1980's:

> Dan Bell is idly watching the Dow-Jones societal wire (formerly the business wire): "Consumer Indignation Index down .04 percent

. . . Back Power Ratio steady . . ." Suddenly Bell calls excitedly, "Mike, Bert, come here quick. The Native Restlessness Index has hit an all-time high!" The advisors go into special session with their staff, then report their conclusions and recommendations to the President, who the next day asks Congress for emergency legislation to install a nationwide network of plastic swimming pools. He activates the National Guard, and calls a White House Conference (27, p. 1038).

The situation in which a conceptual framework intended for use in one context is applied to another has been called by Pirie the Pied Piper Problem, and is exemplified here by the application of techniques of social science or psychiatry to politics. Pirie observed that "the particular type of error with which we are concerned is the transference of a concept into a field in which it is inapplicable; the more useful the concept is in its own field the greater the danger . . . the value of concepts, in their own field, is measurable by the amount of harm they do when it is assumed that they apply in others" (29). Basically, the problem seems to be related to efforts to replace concepts from one field with those of another. A preferred application would be a form of cooperation rather than competitive replacement. The great task facing the social sciences, psychiatry, or any other field of specialization is to correct not the errors and illusions of other sciences or professions but those of its own. This caution is particularly relevant to psychiatry, a field that was isolated for so many years and which has precipitously emerged from its professional isolation onto the arena of social and civil change in the face of such great popular enthusiasm and federal support. This sudden and drastic reversal of role from insular medical practitioner to that of social reformer and shaper of present and future patterns of society is a task requiring as much humility and caution as any other specific characteristic. Particularly in our time, the psychiatrist must be aware of the problem of the philosopher king.

THE THREE DIMENSIONS OF DEPTH

Psychoanalysts traditionally have spoken and written about "depth" in the understanding of mental life. It is characteristically implied if not stated directly that degree of depth—in interpretation, insight, understanding, recollection, and so forth—is an index of talent: the deeper the better. In the language of psychoanalysis, the opposite of deep is surface or superficial, and these labels carry disparaging connotations. The psychoanalytic metaphor of depth is thus bound to value judgments. Such rhetorical qualities make difficult the presentation of other viewpoints, whether neurological or social-psychiatric, since it is implied that such non-analytic thought is inevitably in some way less profound.

Some etymological background will be helpful as a preface to a discussion of the present use of the concept of depth in psychoanalysis. The first known application of the metaphor of depth or profundity to the concept of mind or soul can be traced to an era in Greece between Homer and the Classical Age that is frequently called the "lyric period." Heraclitus and presumably earlier lyric poets used this new figure of speech in reference to intellectual and spiritual matters. Terms such as *deep thinking, deep knowledge, deep pondering, deep pain* came to be common, whereas they were unknown to Homer, who relied on a notion of quantity in such expressions as *much knowledge, many sorrows,* and *countless grief.* Snell attributes Homer's quantitative approach to the fact that he relied totally on visual models. He who has seen much is in fact often knowledgeable; hence Homer relied on "much knowing" (30). The reasons for this switch to a metaphor of depth are worth examining, since its current usage is now responsible for much linguistic confusion in our field. The concept of depth seems to be employed in an effort to say, in a sense, that what is to be understood or described is beyond what the eye can see, that the issues are too complex to use a visual model in which clearly discrete items (i.e., sorrows) can be grouped together like billiard balls and counted.

There is little question that the term *depth* has subsequently assumed rhetorical implications. The psychoanalytic claim that its understanding of mental life is deeper than that provided by other theoretical approaches represents a misuse of the metaphor of depth. If the concept does now function as a spurious form of value judgment, it shall have lost its intended function. If that is the case, we must retire Heraclitus' metaphor as currently meaningless. What was a brilliant departure of the lyric poets—trying to wrest the conceptualization of human processes out of the purely visual—should not be adapted to the promotion of one theoretical approach to the understanding of human behavior at the expense of all alternative theories.

Extracted from its metaphorical framework, the question of depth in psychoanalytic theory is a component of *metapsychology*. In his use of this term, Freud wanted to designate a comprehensive (deep) analysis of an event (mental process) in a way that would include multiple interpretations of it in terms, to paraphrase Jones (31, p. 185), of its *dynamic* attributes, its *topographical* features, and its *economic* significance. The term metapsychology has been widely accepted and extended by followers of Freud. More recently, Rapaport and Gill (32) have argued that a metapsychological discussion must now include five different points of view instead of the initial three posited by Freud. They are the structural (under which topographical is now subsumed), dynamic, economic, genetic, and adaptive. The application of such an exposition to the discussion of a specific problem may be found in Gill and Brenman's review of hypnosis (33). Such points of view represent models, each different, which when put together do indeed represent an impressive and comprehensive battery of "fixes" on any event being studied.

It is generally agreed that Freud was the first to organize his thought in this manner. Jones (31) reports that he first used the term *metapsychology* to mean the study of the assumptions of psychology in 1896 in a letter to Fleiss. Its popularity stems from the twelve papers, usually called the metapsychological papers, that Freud wrote in Vienna during World War I, when his practice declined and he had the chore of keeping two psychoanalytic journals in operation. Additional interest in these papers has been heightened because the last seven were never published and the manuscripts, other than their titles, have not survived.

However, metapsychology and therefore depth are not necessarily relevant exclusively to psychoanalytic theory. Neurological and social psychiatry can be considered within the same frame of reference. If we take "structure" as an example we see that the structure (structural model) that the psychoanalyst thinks of himself as treating consists of id, ego, and superego; for the organically-oriented psychiatrist it is the brain, and for the social psychiatrist a system or natural group such as a family, network or community. A further consideration of social psychiatry in the formal context worked out for psychoanalytic metapsychology provides an introduction to the following chapters. Each chapter takes one of the points of view of metapsychology, or the assumptions underlying pathogenesis and treatment, and expands this theme from the point of view of social psychiatry. It would be possible to do the same for neurological psychiatry, although this task is not here undertaken.

THREE SCHOOLS OF THOUGHT AND THE
METAPSYCHOLOGICAL MODELS

School Model	Organic	Psycho- Analytic	Social Psychiatric
Genetic	Chromosomes	Oral, Anal, Phallic, Genital	Epigenetics
Structural	Brain	Id, Ego, Superego	Networks, Interfaces
Dynamic	Neuro-physiology	Conflict	Cycles, Spirals
Economic	Energy as in physics, chemistry	Libido	"the great chain of life"
Topographical	States of consciousness	Conscious, preconscious, unconscious	Contrite fallibilism
Pathogenesis and diagnosis	A.P.A. Diagnosis Medical Model		Social breakdown syndrome
Treatment	Chemical surgical	Psycho-analysis	"Family" Therapy

The table above illustrates the application of the metapsychological format to the three major schools of psychiatry. In the far left column are four of the five metapsychological categories; across the top are the three schools of thought. In each box of the table is a word or phrase providing an example of what might be discussed under this heading by each school. It can be seen that an equally comprehensive or "deep" analysis of an event in mental life is potentially available from each school of thought. While Freud was the first to clearly conceptualize such an analysis and to name it metapsychology, it is both possible and profitable to organize material within the other two large theoretical groupings in the same manner. For example, in the social area, family homeostasis is an economic concept, the family is a structural model, and the natural history of a marriage uses a genetic model. In the organic area, the brain is a structural model, neurophysiology is a dynamic concept, and the genetic study of schizophrenia can hardly be denied admission as a genetic model.

In the table I have omitted the adaptive point of view usually included in metapsychology and retained the topographical point of view which is now usually subsumed in the structural. Topography is included for heuristic purposes: it gives me an opportunity to discuss at length the unconscious and its alternatives. The adaptive point of view is omitted because I feel that it might be more successfully equated with the entire social psychiatric school of thought—in short, that it belongs to the other axis of the table, next to organic and psychoanalytic. The attempt to assimilate it into psychoanalytic theory rather than see it as independent at a basic level is thus regarded as unproductive.

As I have noted, Rapaport and Gill (32) do not share my view, and treat the adaptive model as a legitimate component of metapsychology. However, they report that questions about its inclusion were raised by almost every reader of the early drafts of their paper:

> Moreover, there are still some psychoanalysts who refuse to recognize that the psychoanalytic theory does imply adaptive assumptions. They equate adaptation with adjustment, and fear that to take adaptive considerations seriously leads inevitably to the course taken by various schools of psychoanalytic thought who employ their enthusiastic discovery of environmental relationships for the purpose of defensive denial of drive and intrapsychic conflict. These psychoanalysts to the contrary notwithstanding, the question is not whether adaptive considerations form a part of psychoanalysis, but rather: Is the adaptive point of view of the same level of abstraction as the others? can it be considered "metapsychological" at all? or can the adaptive propositions of psychoanalysis be satisfactorily derived from

the classical points of view which Freud, in his definition of meta-psychology, conceived of in the context of a *mental event* without reference to environmental relations (32)?

Within the Freudian corpus, I believe that adaptation does not rank as metapsychological but is instead the basis for another point of view. In a sense, this entire book presents this argument. Precisely the opposite occurs with reference to topography. Rapaport and Gill write, "This assumption does not distinguish between conscious and unconscious psychological forces, because that distinction *is not an assumption* but an inference from empirical observations, and is thus a proposition of the special theory of psychoanalysis but not of metapsychology" (32, italics added). In this case social psychiatric theory maintains that the distinction between conscious and unconscious is an assumption. (For an appreciation of this point, it is necessary to read Chapter Four.)

It is at this point that the non-ideological nature of this book, and its corollary, the absence of conflict herein, can be illustrated. In their attempt to deal with metapsychology Rapaport and Gill conclude that the sources they studied "do not fulfill the program implied in Freud's definition. They do not state systematically that minimal set of assumptions on which the psychoanalytic theory rests" (32). The two points made here, that adaptation is not metapsychology and that topography is, are contributed on the basis of a study of a different theoretical program: social psychiatry. In the sense that the fish is the last one to recognize that he is surrounded by water, the psychoanalyst may be the last one to identify the very basic assumptions that create the atmosphere of his theory. It is through the delineation of a contrasting and independent theory that such assumptions begin to stand out in comparison. Accordingly, the author hopes that these essays will be read and found helpful by both psychoanalysts and social psychiatrists.

CHAPTER TWO

Inner and Outer Space: Dynamics

In an early scene of the *Iliad* Achilles is about to attack his comrade-in-arms and commander, Agamemnon, as a result of a sudden and superficial quarrel. The scene has fascinated classicists for generations and now, with the call to reexamine the classical world with the tools of behavioral science, social psychiatrists as well. This passage illustrates two questions which I shall discuss in this chapter. First, why are these men so barbaric; why are they unstable and irrational to the ultimate degree and yet heroes, leaders, and the elite of the period? Second, why is the narrative so crudely interrupted just at this point with what is today a rather silly episode? Achilles, in fact, does not kill Agamemnon because he feels a tug on his hair and, there and then, enters into a logical dialogue with the goddess Athena, who is invisible to all others. She discusses with him the pros and cons of his continuing the fight or delaying immediate gratification for future rewards. Why could it not merely be said that Achilles thought about the matter and decided to hold his temper rather than that he hallucinated Athena, for that is what we would call it today? Athena certainly sounds suspiciously like an ego function: she delays gratification and so forth. A search through the *Iliad* reveals that this scene is not a chance occurrence, but that there is extensive savage and incontinent affect and clumsy external divine machinery, invoked for purposes of restraint. We are here provided with an opportunity to study a completely different dynamic system.

The answers to both questions lie in a study of language. It must be remembered that the report of Achilles' external (rather than internal) dialogue was composed, to the best of our knowledge, in 750 B.C. or earlier. Since that time we have slowly learned to talk about ourselves in different terms, and so we behave differently. In this chapter, one of two devoted to dynamics, I shall review briefly the origin of the concept of inner psychological machinery which replaced that of divine machinery of Bronze Age Greece. Following this, I shall discuss certain criticisms of the basic notions involved in our modern concept as an introduction to a radically new way of talking about human behavior and dynamics that defines social psychiatry. Last, I shall present brief case excerpts of a social psychiatric construct called a *release* that is based on this new approach.

LANGUAGE STRUCTURE: THE MASS NOUN

In our language we have two types of nouns: those nouns denoting individual physical things (like *ant, heart*) and mass nouns, denoting physical things that do not have boundaries (like *water, wood, meat*). Mass nouns lack plurals and in English drop indefinite articles (we say "an ant" but just "water"). The reader may be aware of some exceptions which will not be discussed here; neither will other aspects of the analysis of language structure. In the interest of brevity I shall focus on the mass noun.

Mass nouns are rarely experienced as such by individuals. For instance, water comes in a container most of the time. Thus we have a formula for talking about water; we say "glass of water," "bottle of water," and so forth. This is, of course, obvious. However, when we come to other mass nouns like *wood*, the formula for talking about them (for instance, "stick of wood") does not use an actual container; but it is *as if* "stick" were a container.

Similarly, when we say "drop of water" we are no longer using a container like a glass or a bottle but an "as if" container, an imaginary container. Such a device Whorf referred to as "the binomial formula," a container-ingredient metaphor: "Our language patterns often require us to name a physical thing by a binomial that splits the reference into a formless item plus a form" (1, p. 141).

In our language today we carry this binomial formula still further, especially when we try to describe processes and not things. We have seen that there are two types of containers (real like "bottle" and imaginary like "stick"). We also have two types of ingredients, real and imaginary. In English when we say, "In summer it is hot," we have constructed a sentence with an imaginary container (summer), in which there is an imaginary ingredient (heat). An alternative construction would be, "During summer heat occurs." Heat, we now know, is a process and not a thing. However, the way we phrase or think of things often determines our behavior. For instance, because of the *imaginary* ingredient "heat," scientists as recently as the last century looked for the substance of heat, something they called "caloric." Materials were actually weighed when hot to see if they were heavier. When no result was forthcoming, it was assumed that the scales were not sensitive enough.

For Newtonian dynamics to be used efficiently it is necessary to have substances created in this metaphorical fashion. For instance, when we conceive of a wave of water as a container with content that travels from one place to another, we can measure its speed, acceleration, direction, and so forth. However, when we try to express the fact that a wave is not actually a thing that stands by itself and travels, but a disturbance of a medium (no water, it must be remembered, actually moves the length of the wave's travel) we have a difficult abstract process, almost insurmountable in English and other Indo-European languages. What we do in English to use these dynamics is to "objectify" processes, to make a container-ingredient thing of a process (1). The importance of this will become apparent below when interpersonal processes are discussed.

EARLY GREEK THOUGHT

Early Bronze-Age Greek man first thought of himself without using mass nouns or the binomial formula. That is, he thought of himself as the juxtaposition of individual nouns: arms, legs, the heart, lungs, and so forth. Snell (2) discusses this with reference to Greek "geometric" art, in which human figures actually look like parts put together at joints rather than a whole. *Soma* meant only dead body, self-reference was by name, and skin was about as close as one could get to our concept of body.

With the advent of new mass nouns (for example, *flesh*) it was necessary to invent new containers (*body*). At this point in the development of the topography of early Greek man we have an imaginary container in which there are mass mouns. It is hard to realize that *body* was not always used as a concept, yet *body*, like *drop* or *stick*, cannot actually stand without its contents and is "imaginary," whereas an actual container, for instance *skin*, can stand empty. At this stage, man talked of himself as we talk today of a "stick of wood" or a "drop of water." There was no spiritual area divorced from the corporeal. Hence, man thought of his actions as resulting from changes in his organic contents (the mass nouns). *Vapor* was a particularly popular mass noun, and vaporous changes were thought to cause behavioral changes. Although we now know this is wrong medically, real vapor, such as that which appears to come from the body when we breathe on a cold day, was being referred to when early Greek man talked of vaporous changes.

Just as there was a different concept of the individual, there was a different concept of the community. The group or community was thought of as having a soul which belonged to the God-King. The well-being of the community was considered as deriving from that of the king. Regicide, therefore, was an act of destruction against the whole tribe. To a certain extent this tribal dependency on the king appears to have been related to the scarcity of vital resources such as bronze armor and chariots, tools, information exchange, and commerce, which only the privileged few could utilize. For survival purposes it was thus necessary to depend on those who did possess them. The social ferment that followed a change in this distribution (with the advent of the Phoenician alphabet, coined money, cheap and plentiful iron) was extraordinary. The warlord was no longer necessary. But until the time when commerce, weapons, and writing were available to all, there existed this group cohesion—not only *in fact* but in the way people thought about themselves, *in their psychology*.

The person, conceived of as entirely physical, belonged to the state. Just as we would not credit a little finger with individuality of soul or decision, so the person was not credited with it in early Greece. Man was not seen as one who could initiate any deliberate actions, nor, for that matter, did gods appear often to help him do so. The tribe led by the king was said to be the exclusive executive organ. There were no provisions *in the psychology* for modern, executive functioning by the individual. Men were led to believe they were essentially reactors, not initiators. This led to an individual who was savage and impulsive, by our standards. In the rare event that individual reflection and hesitation occurred —for instance when Achilles, although fuming, does not draw his sword on Agamemnon—it cannot be expressed as an inner dialogue (that is, as his doing) but is seen as an imaginary outer dialogue: Athena appears to him, pulls his hair, and warns him of the danger of fighting with Agamemnon. This is not just a figure of speech used for color. The author cannot say, "He holds his temper" (notice that *that* figure of speech "objectifies" a process by making *temper* a noun), or that Athena "gets his attention." Much of the narrative of the *Iliad* is, for us, interrupted by the appearance of gods, whose presence was used to express the rare situations when thought occurs. When it came to explaining further what happened in the outer dialogue, the god was said to literally add (breathe in) some vaporous mass noun to the contents of the body. Thus we still have with us the term *inspired*. At this time it was taken literally (3).

THE CHANGE TO MODERN THOUGHT

It was a group of rebellious poets (Sappho, Anacreon, Archilochus, and those unknowns preceding them) who departed from this conception of man and community. They still retained the older notions for unusual or violently discontinuous events (like our present use of the term *inspired*) but they attributed to themselves the ability to act as agents of their own thoughts and feelings. To do this they had to revise their way of thinking about themselves—their psychology. They now spoke of a content of themselves which was not physical or corporeal but clearly spiritual. There was now an inner life which was more important (to the individual) than the outer community life. Archilochus was able to write poetry celebrating the saving of his own life in battle because he could justify it in terms of conserving his inner life, which did not belong to the state and was not expendable.[1] Before this a soldier (whether or not he also wrote poetry) was to return "with his shield or on it." Archilochus celebrates his cowardliness because his concept of an inner life, belonging to the individual, freed him from the bondage to the god-king.

The content of this inner life was now conceptualized as imaginary mass nouns like *caloric*, constructed on the model of changing an individual noun (a *heart*) to a metaphor (he has "heart"). These or similar devices have subsequently been used for centuries. For instance, a choking sensation (*angoise* in French) became *anxiety* (5). The dynamics of these nouns became responsible for behavior.

Another device was to take the outer dialogue and turn that, too, into an imaginary mass noun. For instance, the demon *Phobus* became *fear*, a substance seen as inside us as an "affect." With the advent of imaginary mass nouns there was a need for a new container. It was clear that fear, for instance, could not be inside a *body*. The new container I shall call "inner space." The ultimate achievement of Classical Greek civilization was the development of this mode of self-reference. We live as we do thanks to it. It was to this idea that Freud added his concept of the unconscious along the same metaphorical lines. His was not a radical departure but the addition of an extra container in our imaginary inner space for that which was "unconscious'd." This was necessary, Freud argued, to more effectively explain our behavior. As Rieff (6) has pointed out, it also has influenced our individ-

1.   Some lucky Thracian has my noble shield.
            I had to run; I dropped it in a wood.
            But I got clear away, Thank God. So hang
            The shield! I'll get another, just as good (4, p. 88).

ual and political behavior. It created an ideal which Rieff calls "psychological man." In many ways it continues the trajectory established by the Greeks when they broke away from the tremendous pressures of society imposed on them in the Bronze Age by certain conditions of life and their concept of themselves. Freud freed man even further—from the bondage of the family, religion, morality, guilt, and so forth. By being essentially anti-superego and pro-insight, psychoanalysis has, according to Rieff, allowed the rich to lower the pressures of communal purpose upon themselves even further. The population implosion and modern technology have, however, created such pressures again. It is therefore necessary to rethink our dynamic psychology.

CRITICISM OF INNER SPACE

In the Soviet Union, Great Britain, and the United States there have been three major movements critical of the concept of inner space. They were all extremely active in the 1930's, although they apparently had no contact with each other. Consequently, each developed its own vocabulary and style of criticism. However, there is a remarkable agreement among them as to the alternative in behavioristic terms to that which they criticize. In addition, each school focuses on some aspect of communication in its criticism.

The Soviet criticism appears to stem from overt political needs. The whole notion of a collective society as envisioned in the U.S.S.R. requires a concept of man with whom the State has a right to be actively and intimately involved. The "psychological man" whom Rieff describes would be a political criminal in the Soviet system. It is for this reason that *Dr. Zhivago*, Pasternak's novel of a Russian individualist, was banned. It behooved Soviet psychologists in the 1930's to find alternatives to Western psychology. As Luria and Leontiev put it: "The first and most important task in that time consisted in freeing oneself, on the one hand from vulgar behaviorism, and on the other from the subjective approach to mental phenomenon as exclusively inner subjective conditions which can only be investigated introspectively" (7).

Under this pressure Pavlov turned from conditioning to a

study of communication—which he relabeled the "secondary signaling system." Vygotsky (7) produced a brilliant series of studies challenging the notion that thought was anything more than inhibited dialogue, by showing its development in children from "accompanying speech" (Piaget's "egocentric speech"). The result was to demonstrate the social nature and origins of consciousness, dynamics, and intellect and deny the Western concept of consciousness and intellect as existing in a special realm, inner space, in which the State could not properly be involved.

British criticism of the concept of inner space has been called Analytic or Linguistic Philosophy. The origin of this school of thought is generally connected with Ludwig Wittgenstein, who previously was associated with Logical Positivism. His own story of how he began to think along lines that were critical of inner space concepts is distinctly non-political. He said that he frequently talked about his notion that language was a picture of reality with an Italian economist (Piero Sraffa) who one day gestured to him with a classical Neopolitan expression of contempt and demanded to know of what that was a picture. Wittgenstein took the criticism to heart. He did not spell out how he arrived at his final position from this gesture, and for all we know, the story is apocryphal. However, it is possible in the interest of exposition to supply a route by which this can be achieved. Wittgenstein became interested in verbal gestures like "Aha!" "Hurrah!" and so forth. These gestures do not depict anything, as we know, but are merely *indexes* of a certain state of the individual expressing them. Wittgenstein's radical insight was to liken other verbal utterances such as "Now I understand" (which seems to imply or offer a picture of an inner process of understanding) to expressions like "Hurrah!" He denied that either "Hurrah!" or "Now I understand" was a picture of something. He argued further that the whole idea of inner processes was based on the incorrect assumption that language is a picture of reality, which had been so strikingly upset with Sraffa's contemptuous gesture. The school of "philosophical psychology" called British Linguistic Philosophy that developed from these unusual beginnings became extremely critical of the concept of inner space by considering, as Wittgenstein had, the misuses of language. An example of a linguistic analysis of the phrase, "I don't remember" will be presented below.

In the late 1920's Harry Stack Sullivan and William Alanson White, under the auspices of the American Psychiatric Association, convened conferences in an effort to integrate the social sciences with psychiatry. As reviewed in Chapter One, many of the issues raised in the Soviet Union and England had been dealt with simultaneously or even earlier by American pragmatists and social psychologists in different terminology and from different motives. C. Wright Mills, himself often classified as a pragmatist, reviewed the complex origins of this thinking in his Ph.D. thesis (8). In brief, he saw it as stemming from the change in the original religious nature of higher education in America created by the need for applied scientists and the efforts of such men living in two worlds (scientific and moral) to maintain their values by integrating science, philosophy, psychology, and morals. The similarity between social psychology and Wittgenstein's position can be demonstrated by this quote from G.H. Mead: "Language does not simply symbolize a situation or object which is already there in advance; it makes possible the existence or the appearance of that situation or object, for it is part of the mechanisms whereby it . . . is created" (9, p. 189). The difference between linguistic philosophy and social psychology is that the former has restricted itself to criticisms of the creations of language, its practitioners acting like physicians toward what they deemed pathological developments, whereas social psychology has been more intrigued with the description of the process by which these mythical structures like inner space have been developed. It was this latter movement that Sullivan and White succeeded in introducing into psychiatry.

The only alternative to the metaphors of inner space has been called, unfortunately, *behaviorism*. As we have seen in the Soviet statement, "vulgar behaviorism" is nobody's ideal program. Watsonian behaviorism had so many defects that to speak of it as the current position of any group is to create a straw man. However, the term is well established. G. H. Mead, a social psychologist, was forced reluctantly to use the term about himself as was Ryle, the dean of British philosophers, probably in both cases because of its greater familiarity than *social psychology*. It appears, however, that, as social psychiatric thought becomes well known and clearly differentiated from organic and psychoanalytic thought, it will be unnecessary to emphasize that the alternative to "inner space" and its dynamics is inevitably "outer space" and that what this outer space "contains" is behavior.

As Chappell has reviewed, there are four ways in which "vulgar (Watsonian) behaviorism" has been refined (10, pp. 11–12). First, there are *dispositions* to behave in addition to observable acts. Anger, for instance, is defined as a disposition to behave in a certain way, much like the concept of brittleness, which is also a disposition to certain behavior. (A brittle glass is disposed to break.) Neither anger nor brittleness need be seen as inside a person or thing. Second, the notion of behavior itself is modified to refer, not to movement, but activity. Fighting, for instance, is not the mechanical repetition of a specific movement but an *activity* which might even be accomplished by silent, withdrawn non-movement. Third, such activity is set in a social setting, within a social system, as an integral part of the behavior. Anger cannot be truly defined without considering the standards of a social group; what is anger in one setting is not in another. As G. H. Mead has said, "Social psychology studies the activity or behavior of the individual as it lies within the social process; the behavior of an individual can be understood only in terms of the behavior of the whole social group of which he is a member, since his individual acts are involved in larger, social acts which go beyond himself and which implicate the other members of that group (9, pp. 133–134)." A fourth refinement is to accept first-person statements as legitimate data that may constitute a final authority in some circumstances with regard to mental phenomena. This last point has been added because behavior is the final common pathway for many starting points. Teeth-grinding may be anger or the result of a seizure, sudden standing up may be the result of a leg cramp or impatience. Facial expressions may be a function of anger or a stomach ache. In most actual situations, therefore, the individual has *more* data than the investigator, not data of a privileged, theoretically different nature, and it is practical to ask for it. With these four important refinements it becomes possible to talk about behavior without using inner space metaphors or having to accept the crude behaviorism of Watson.

PRACTICAL APPLICATIONS IN THERAPY

Without concepts of inner space, the dynamics we must discuss are considerably modified. It is not my intention to discuss treatment at great length but to illustrate, using a series of interview fragments, that from the point of view of social psychiatry several options that differ from those of more traditional models are available.

Because the term *behaviorism* has been used, it must first be differentiated from the so-called behavior therapies and from what is to follow. Conditioning and learning theory have been applied to symptoms of individuals, with reported success. Thus a child apparently can be helped to stop wetting the bed through the use of electrical equipment which wakes him up just as he starts to be enuretic. This is *not* the type of therapy referred to here. However, if we use this example of behavior therapy in which the child stops wetting the bed, it is possible to make a transition to that which shall be discussed. Suppose that another older child in the family who had never been enuretic now started to wet the bed. Even if the same equipment is used again with this older child, it would be appropriate to study the pathology of the family system. In this family there seems to be a repetitive pattern, a rule, that someone has to wet the bed. In treatment it may be necessary to change the group rule, to *release* people from it, in addition to dealing with individual symptoms.

In the three case excerpts presented below, an effort shall be made to present a glimpse of what therapy is like without concepts of inner space. These three excerpts are presented because they deal with one phenomenon that I have termed a "release." In no situation did the therapist attempt to explain memories or the report of events in terms of what was happening inside the individual. Instead, a social process, a release, was focused on and manipulated. If, however, a therapist were to use the concepts of inner space, he would rely on dynamic notions or what Ryle prefers to call "paramechanical notions" (since they deal with happenings in inner space that do not actually correspond to anything in the world of physics). These para-mechanical notions deal with forces on inner imaginary objects, repression, suppression, blocks, and so forth. They are manipulated in psychoanalysis by concentration on the individual patient and the use of "aids to memory" such as dream interpretation, free association, and transference. As we have seen in the first part of this chapter, the use of mechanics in a situation of this sort could be predicted from the tendency of the binomial formula to objectify processes into "things" or thing-like forms. Without the binomial formula this method of talking about patients is not possible.

Case One (Family Therapy)

Therapist: (to younger brother) What did Mr. H. (co-therapist) just say?
Child: I dunno.
Therapist: Do you always sit like that? Head down?
Child: No. (smiles)
Therapist: O.K., sit up. Look at your mother. . . .
(to mother) Is it all right if he says what he heard?
Mother: Sure.
Therapist: (to child) Tell us.
Child: (proceeds to report what he heard)

Comments:

This brief dialogue is offered here as an introduction to the concept of a license or release. In this rather innocuous dialogue, the child "remembers" after he is released or licensed to do so by his mother. ("Is it all right if he says what he heard?") In this case, the therapist easily structures the situation so that the release may be given.

Case Two (Family Therapy)

Therapist: Now, is it all right for Stanley to say why he wants to go to the hospital?
Mother: Sure, he can tell you about how poor we are and.
. . .
Stanley: (no comment)
Therapist: No, that's not doing it. You have to release him to talk about anything, not give him a subject. Go ahead, tell him it's all right.
Mother: Go ahead, Stanley, what's wrong? You know the trouble in the streets. . . .

Stanley:	(no comment)
Therapist:	No. Again, try again. It may not be "trouble in the streets."
Mother:	O.K.
Therapist:	Are you sure it's O.K.? Tell Stanley if it is.
Mother:	Stanley, it's O.K. to say anything that's true.
Stanley:	(no comment)
Therapist:	No. No. No. It's too confusing trying to decide what you mean by "what is true." Just let him say what he's feeling.
Mother:	Stanley, these people want to know what you're feeling.
Stanley:	(no comment)
Therapist:	No. Wrong again. That's four times. You have to say that *you* want him to tell you what's wrong. Can he say what's wrong *at home? With you?*
Mother:	(with feeling) Stanley, for heaven's sake, will you tell me what's wrong at home.
Stanley:	Cooking. . . .
Therapist:	(to mother) Good. That's one thing. But Stanley's old enough to speak in sentences. . . . (etc.)

Comment:

The technical difficulties are demonstrated here with the subtle way the mother was able to appear to be following the request of the therapist and yet not licensing the patient to discuss his real problems. Incidentally, the session was quite instructive to the mother, who had perceived herself, as had many others, as a weak, "overwhelmed," sick (schizophrenic) person. She left the session considering the question (raised by her) of whether she weren't a tyrant, controlling other people.

Case Three (Diagnostic Interview)

Young girl:	I had a convulsion.
Therapist:	I know, but I'm not that kind of doctor. I don't know about convulsions. I know about feelings and thoughts. What happened just before this thing?
Young girl:	I don't remember. All my life I've been having convulsions and they'd call the ambulance. I'd wake up later.

Therapist: I know you don't remember now, I believe you, really. But you can remember if you try. I'm sure you don't even know what I'd be interested in hearing about. Tell me where you were, where you were standing, for instance.

Young girl: (Proceeds to tell of feeling terrible about enlisting in the military, feeling overcome with nausea and deciding that it would help if she went into the bathroom to vomit, where she had the "happy thought": if only everything would go black.)

Comment:

In this case the medical setting of a clinic suggests certain "rules" of reporting events. The therapist licensed other "memories."

The concept of a release as a social dynamic is in direct conflict with the dynamic mechanisms of inner space that are said to operate in the unconscious. If we utilize Chappell's four points about modern behaviorism reviewed above, we can see that a release is a behavioristic concept.

First, the therapist's concern for dispositions prompts him to think about the conditions that dispose people to act. An amnesia in Case Three is seen not as a block in inner space but as the result of disposing factors. The patient is not disposed to report certain events unless the "cognitive map" or "demand characteristics" of the situation favor it.

Second, the therapist concentrates on behavior and activity rather than introspection. Rather than offering an interpretation, he offers one family member a task like "Tell Stanley such and such" in order to release the other family member. One of the assumptions behind the social psychiatrist's use of a task is that an interpretation such as "You are threatened by Stanley's criticism of you because of such and such" (addressed to the same individual) has buried within it essentially the same task of releasing the other person to be critical. Its success depends on social activity, not inner space mechanics.

Third, the setting of the problem, the natural group in which it occurs, is also taken into account. Inner space is, of course, limited to one individual; outer space is not. It is now common to refer to the individual with symptoms as the "index" of group pathology rather than the "patient."

Fourth, the sincere effort to obtain data from patients like Stanley is motivated by the assumption that he is in a position to supply important material that otherwise would have to be obtained over a long period of time. It is not that he has some special privileged access to his inner space and therefore unique data but simply that if he didn't talk about his mother's cooking, or more precisely her lack of it, the time and expense of finding out about this "secret" would be excessive.

A closer look at the case excerpts presented above reveals that they all refer to remembering. In two cases the patient says outright "I don't remember," and in the third, Stanley says nothing at all, thus raising the question "Does he remember?"

The inner space notion associated with remembering is that it essentially consists of "seeing with the mind's eye" or "hearing in the head" a replica of that which is being remembered. The action that goes on in psychotherapy is also conceptualized as going on in the same place—the same inner motion picture screen—as the remembering. Thus this notion would propose that in the cases presented here, the patient remembered when certain things happened in his inner space—let us say "a resistance was removed." What then followed was a showing of the event on what is sometimes called the "phenomenological field." We, of course, recognize this as highly metaphorical speech. No one has seen, or is likely to ever see, the mind's eye.

How can we talk about these processes in more precise terms? It is important to note that *remembering* is often used in two senses: First, it may be used as a synonym for *knowing*. "I remember how to ride a bike" is essentially the same as "I know how to ride a bike." The same can be said for verbal tasks: "I remember (know how to say) the alphabet." In a second sense it is used to certify a past event. The word *remembering* in this sense means a first-hand report of an action. "John hit Mary" and "I remember John hitting Mary" are different in that we are expressing in the later phrase a "certification" of sorts of the former (11). It describes how we have the information, and suggests that we are sure of it. Other languages, such as Hopi, have other ways of describing the source of information.

With this background we can try to understand what the utterance "I don't remember" means. We can see that it refers to a complex of meanings:

1. *I cannot perform that task* (I do not know how, I do not remember)
   a. because I am incapable of it. (For example, although John has seen the Russian alphabet, he does not remember (know) how to say it.)
   b. because I am not licensed or released by my intimates. (For example, Joe does not remember the Russian alphabet because to do so would show an untoward interest in "the commies.")

2. *I cannot be called as a witness* (I don't remember, I can't recall)
   a. because I am incapable of it. (Mary doesn't remember her birth.)
   b. because I am not released. (Margaret does not remember what her mother and brother were fighting about in front of her because it is clear that nobody wants to be reminded of a painful experience.)

A basic confusion occurs in therapy through not distinguishing between the performance of a task and the witnessing of an event. The reconstruction of forgotten experiences is not witnessing but the performance of a complex linguistic task.

Freud writes: "The mechanism of our assistance is easy to understand: we give the patient the conscious anticipatory idea and he then finds the repressed unconscious idea in himself on the basis of its similarity to the anticipatory one. This is the intellectual help which makes it easier for him to overcome the resistances between conscious and unconscious" (12, pp. 141–142). The idea of reconstruction may be replaced with the notion that it is necessary to supply language to an individual in order to make possible the existence or appearance of a situation or object. However, with the "conscious anticipatory idea" (expressed in language) the reality is shaped selectively, as is the moral and political climate.

Another set of confusions develops through not distinguishing between a patient who is bound (not released) and one who is incapable. Interesting and absurd results may be obtained. Thus dianetics, using the techniques of therapists for obtaining releases, began in the 1950's to claim that people could remember (be witnesses to) their birth and intrauterine life. This was based on the notion that cells had memories in them. The metaphor of inner space was merely extended slightly into the cells themselves in order to explain such recall. Equally implausible are the claims of hypnotists to obtain such performances as age-regression (by demonstrating infantile plantar reflexes).

CONCLUSION

The divine machinery of Greece, the inner mechanisms of psychology, and the social psychiatric emphasis on the exchange of behavior within a family or some other natural group are more than just abstract descriptions. They are "ascriptions" (13) in the sense that they do not merely describe a preexisting human condition but are integral moving forces in the making of a state of affairs; they encourage certain meanings and forms of behavior. The author of the *Iliad* had to envisage a god tugging on Achilles' hair to explain a change in his behavior. Much later this event was explained by private dynamic changes in a very special realm, here called inner space. The effect of the newer concept was to change the behavior of men toward each other. It was now easier to hesitate, to initiate, and to come to decisions on one's own. The effect was also to detribalize man.

With the advent of new pressures a distinct third point of view emerges which can be said to suggest that dynamics occur in outer space, in the very same place where people behave. It also asserts that our behavior is not a two-stage affair, first an inner process and then behavior, but rather a single entity. To understand behavioral patterns it is not necessary to pry into supposed hidden performances which maintain or change these patterns on the secret stage of the inner life of the individual. When we adhere to the two-stage approach where a process in one place is presumed to influence actions in another place, we are using essentially the old models of dynamics strongly influenced by a Newtonian concept of forces acting at great distances, such as gravity. The same criticism can be levelled at the notion of divine machinery in ancient Greece. It too spoke of dynamics in one place influencing actions in another. In that case the inner space was the invisible world of the gods, to which special access was allowed by a selected profession, the priests, and outer space was the public, visible world of everyday mortals.

Once it is acknowledged that the actions of an individual *are* the psychology of that individual, what should be made of the various specific dynamic forces previously assigned to his inner space? What alternatives are there to inner affects such as anger? Such issues constitute the subject of the following chapter.

Before concluding this discussion, we might inquire into the political or moral consequences of the new point of view, the one-stage conception of behavior. It has been mentioned that for the Greeks, people were regarded as part of the state. For inner psychology, people were seen as unique entities, emancipated from the demands of citizenship to the point where they no longer felt obliged to consider common interests or social needs. For inner psychology, civilization was an enemy, an intrusive force, and analysis was supposed to make you less of a "good" person. The new point of view, developed in psychiatry by Sullivan and in philosophy by Dewey, is in diametric opposition to the foregoing; it espouses a sense of community, a need for participation in social groupings, which becomes a criterion of adjustment and mental health. Here then is the possibility of dealing with the increasing tribalization of our urbanized world, the forced association with other people, by emphasizing that the quality of such association rather than freedom from it determines one's level of adaptation. In this view, personality does not exist in two worlds, one private and one public, but in one public world where social participation is valued and encouraged.

CHAPTER THREE

Heat,
Electricity,
and Love:
Dynamics

It is not easy to deal scientifically with feelings.
One may attempt to describe their physiological
signs. Where that is impossible . . . nothing remains but to turn to the ideational content
which most readily associates itself with the feeling.

SIGMUND FREUD

As recently as the nineteenth century there
existed in scientific thought the paradoxical notion of a group
of weightless substances or entities called "the imponderables,"
an apt term which simultaneously implied both their weightless-
ness (from *ponderation:* to have weight) and their essential mystery (from the idiom *to weigh in mind*). "It is the imponderab-
bles," mused Oliver Wendell Holmes in a hopeless moment in
1858, "heat, electricity and love that rule the world" (1, p. 352).
This chapter deals predominantly with the last of these impon-

derables and the family of concepts from which it comes. After a brief discussion of historic parallels between heat, electricity, and affect, I shall review some recent attempts to conceptualize affect as a process rather than a substance, an approach that also has historic parallels in the fate of the other two imponderables.

IMPONDERABLES

For the most part, imponderables were conceived as weightless fluids. Holmes' first reference is to caloric, the imponderable substance of heat, which was thought to be squeezed like juice out of the depths of a material when it became hot—for instance, when a metal bar became hot from being pounded by a hammer. In this frame of reference, caloric was somehow said to reside inside the metal bar on some other sort of occult plane. In a manner of speaking, there was a caloric "mind" inside the "body" of everyday things. Eventually this notion was challenged by the mechanical concept of heat, which in Rumford's words (1, p. 347) was viewed as "a kind of motion"—that is, a function of the state of the matter, a property of the behavior of the "body" rather than the "mind." Without reviewing the exciting history of the early pioneers, I would like to point out that the mechanical concept of heat was a difficult conceptual leap. When a metal bar became hot from pounding, one had to believe that particles of the metal began to move faster. As I have said, caloric itself has been rejected as a legitimate concept. The reader knows that heat is a *process,* and he does not feel personally involved in holding a questionable view. As reviewed in Chapter Two, Whorf speaks of this incorrect view, exemplified here by caloric, as the "objectification" of a process by the employment of a linguistic device which he refers to as the "binomial theorem" (a container-ingre dient metaphor; caloric, in this case, is the ingredient). To our surprise, although we reject the concept of caloric today, Whorf has caught us frequently referring to an imponderable heat that is built into the structure of our language.

Electricity, Holmes' second imponderable, was first conceptualized as two occult fluids carrying either plus or minus charges which collected around objects. Electricity fluid, like caloric, was eventually replaced by "a kind of motion" too, but this time as the behavior of the field—that is, as an electromagnetic wave. To quote Maxwell: "Physical science . . . has now . . . entered on the next stage of progress—that in which the energy of a material system is conceived as determined by the configuration and *motion of that system*" (2; italics mine).

About love, Holmes' third imponderable, much more has been written than about heat or electricity, both of which succumbed on analysis to being "a kind of motion." To the extent that love is thought to cause something to happen, to be an occult force that affects an individual (or, more hopefully, two individuals), and that cannot be measured or weighed, we use love as an imponderable and make statements about a fluid-like phenomenon that, like electricity seen as an imponderable, attaches itself to objects and is to be found in a container, the mind.

It was Freud who drew the comparison between love and electricity to its fullest extent. His treatment of affects used an imponderable called *libido*. His concept is explained in the "Defence Neuropsychoses" as, "something having all the attributes of a quantity—although we possess no means of measuring it—a something which is capable of increase, decrease, displacement, and discharge, and which extends itself over the memory traces of an idea *like an electric charge over the surface of the body*" (3, p. 75; italics mine). In other words, libido is something that is similar to caloric and imponderable electricity, which "cathects" an object ("when we are in love a considerable amount of narcissistic libido overflows on to the object" (4, p. 74)). While caloric was seen as an occult juice that was squeezed out of objects, electricity has been likened to an occult butter which spreads itself over the surface of an object. In Freud's concept we have the same type of occult "spread" (libido) which extends over the surfaces in question, only this time the surfaces (ideas) are hidden from view. In Freud's economic theory it is this attachment of the imponderable that creates affects, and its conversion to organic physiological energy that creates structural changes in physiology. This form of explanation was used to consider hysteria, and, as late as 1926, to discuss physiological change in anxiety, which Freud regarded as the normal prototype of hysteria (5, p. 19).

The alternative explanation, to be endorsed here, is the abandonment of the imponderable affect as representative of an entity or substance; instead, affects will be treated as aspects of complex social processes. From the point of view of intellectual history, it is noteworthy that this alternative is, in formal terms, the same substitute for an imponderable seen in the previous discussions of heat and electricity; "a kind of motion"—in this case the motion inherent in the conduct of people with each other.

The approach that treats affect (this time using anxiety as an example) as a property of a social system always evokes the immediate rebuttal that anxiety is associated with physiological change; therefore it cannot be a process in the air between people. It is *not* my aim to deny that bodily changes occur during emotions. Instead, it is with the concept of emotion as a cause that disagreement arises. To present the argument epigrammatically: When I run there are also physiological changes, yet I do not use this fact to support the existence of an imponderable fluid that attaches itself to my organs or muscles or floats around inside me in some occult container to produce fatigue. Running seems a sufficient explanation of my physiological state. In like manner the physiological changes associated with anxiety, love, and so forth are sufficiently explained by the behavior in which the individual participates.

By failing to make a clear, categorical distinction between an isolated sensation (such as a noxious stimulus) and the meaning assigned to the stimulus (discomfort, anxiety, pain), our language has confused us. Much of the objection to affects as system properties stems from an assimilation in our language of many different ingredients under the label "feeling," including physiological reactions to stimuli and consensual assignment of meaning to the stimuli. "Pain," for example, is not a direct index of a noxious stimulus, or else it would be impossible to explain the mitigation of suffering and discomfort by prefrontal leucotomy, opiates, and hypnosis. As Barber pointed out, these last mentioned devices influence the response rather than the felt stimulus (6). The patient's readiness or disposition to respond to the stimulus is modified, not the physiological reaction, and this is partly determined by linguistic phenomena and the attitudes they engender. The discomfort of pain is not inevitably connected with some noxious stimulus although, roughly speaking, there is usually some association. However, the same noxious stimulus can be for one person "extremely painful" and for another "nothing."

AFFECT AS "A KIND OF MOTION"

One can say that we learn about our emotions essentially in the same way that other people learn about them: by observation of conduct. We have more data about ourselves but it is not qualitatively different from that which others gather about us. Bedford has written, "I do not believe that we either do, or should, take anyone's protestations that, for instance . . . he loves his wife, if his conduct offers no evidence whatsoever that he does" (7, p. 116). In short, this argument states that someone who has a specific affect, for example, someone who loves, is one who acts or might act lovingly, not who "feels" a special inner "state." To this basic position Ryle (8, p. 15) adds a "dispositional" concept of emotional words in order to clarify the fact that affects refer to potential as well as current conduct. To say that someone is angry is like saying, "the glass is brittle." The brittle glass is *disposed* to break. It does not have brittleness inside it as an imponderable. Similarly, the angry person is disposed to act in an angry manner. He does not have anger inside him as an imponderable.

Furthermore, what constitutes an angry manner is determined by consensus—that is, there must be people who judge that a given kind of behavior or disposition is to be called anger (7). The same applies to anxiety or any other emotion. There is no absolute standard by which one can measure whether an action is to be defined as anxious; it must be agreed upon, and therefore is a phenomenon relative to a specific context of judges. When I say that I am anxious, I am saying that I have empirical evidence suggesting that I am disposed to behave in a certain way that I and my peers have decided to call anxiety. Above all I am not reporting the occurrence of a new category of imponderable events or mental acts going on inside me. Working with couples and families in psychotherapy, I have often encountered instances where certain conduct (e.g., anger) in one social or familial context is not so regarded in another. This is most clearly shown when a member of one family marries a member of another family which has an entirely different system for codifying affects. Thus, what is "anger," as diagnosed by tone of voice, body posture, word selection, and so forth by one group, would be labeled by someone from a different vantage point as, for instance, a way of making a point, or normal problem-solving, or even affection.

LABELING AS SOCIAL ACTION

"Having" an emotion is not a subcutaneous fact; it is a type of transaction. Such human activity has been analyzed in terms of two levels: the conduct itself, and commentary about that conduct. Classically this commentary has been regarded as neutral and separate from the behavior itself. Sullivan (9, p. 14) challenged this notion with his concept of "participant observer," Bateson (10) with his "double-bind" hypothesis, Dewey (11) with a discussion of the transactional significance of naming, and G. H. Mead (12) with his concept of "meaning." In addition, Hart (13) has been careful to use the term *ascribe* rather than *describe;* we "ascribe" an emotion when we label it. By using this term it is clear that the transaction involved in labeling an emotion is more active than "describing"; it is similar to the giving, assigning, or bestowing (of meaning) and is not merely revealing the appearance, nature, and attributes of a preexisting imponderable substance.

Another way of making this distinction—that the labeling of an affect is an integral part of the conduct of the affect itself and not simply parallel commentary about it—is to say that the assignment of meaning is a "performatory statement." A performatory statement is one that does not describe or name but is in itself an action (14). To recite a marriage vow is to do more than make a statement; it is to get involved in a specific transaction. To vow in that sense is performatory. Similarly the statement, "I'll take this one," when asked to make a choice is not a descriptive statement but a major part of choosing. The value of this distinction is readily seen when applied to psychotherapy. For example, the girl who thinks of herself as "loving" her parents will continue to act the way she does. However, on encountering and accepting a different set of labels—for instance, that she is not the good daughter who loves her parents but instead is seen as hopelessly involved in an oedipal situation (with the affects that implies), dominated by her superego, prudish, and dull—her behavior will change. Both interpretations of her behavior are profoundly involved with the action itself; they are performatory. They are ascriptions, not descriptions.

HOW LABELING CONFLICTS ARE SOLVED

Emotional labels, then, are "interpretations" of transactions, providing we have a revised concept of these interpretations as a very significant part of the behavioral events themselves. Combining the various points made above, it may be said that emotions resemble many legal and moral judgments that have been referred to by Hart (13) as "defeasible." A defeasible concept is a highly variable interpretation of conducts by particular people within their given frame of reference. Studying how such an interpretation becomes fixed, Hart and others have concluded that it is accepted only if all other alternatives are defeated—that is, by negative proof. Such interpretations or concepts are called defeasible. Murder, for example, is a judgment that is established by defeating the alternative explanations, one of which is accident; mental illness is established by defeating the alternatives of eccentricity or poor judgment (15). Since many of the notions that are found, on analysis, to be defeasible are regarded by the general public as established on the basis of truth, justice, or medical fact, the concept is a difficult one for many people to accept. They rightly suspect that it undermines quite a few of their notions of how things work in their social world. It is much more comfortable to believe that murder, for instance, is an actual fact decided on a true-false basis than to see it as the interpretation by particular people at a given time that is perfectly capable of reinterpretation in changed contexts. As indicated above, the same is true about mental illness; this label too is an interpretation of events and not a medical certainty, as Szasz (16) and Goffman (17) have shown.

RELEVANCE TO PSYCHOTHERAPY

This combative notion of how a defeasible concept is established derives from previous points made here: affects are conduct, dispositions, relative to a given social system, and performatory. They do not refer to absolutes, but represent the interpretive judgments of the observer which cannot be regarded as right or wrong per se. If two people or families or groups differ in their frames of reference regarding the meaning of behavior, these differences could not be resolved by appeal to a third party or by negotiation. Each group would be entitled to refer all events to its frame of reference, its social system, its family. For example, how is it possible to decide whether or not a husband should beat his wife? I will assume that most readers come from a frame of reference where this is taboo and would signify one particular affect to them. Suppose, however, that a husband from this frame of reference married a wife from a frame of reference where it was believed that husbands beat their wives *if they love them*. It is impossible to settle this difference in such a way that both beliefs coexist; one must be defeated. It is, of course, possible for the disagreement to be dealt with through avoidance. However, to the extent that a common task were required of these two people, each from a different system, there would be endless difficulty until one interpretation triumphed over the other. Such concepts are defeasible. Quite clearly they, and the conduct associated with them, are not merely trimmings but vital aspects of the performance, the very glue of the transaction.

If it is true that we are dealing with aspects of conduct and not imponderable forces, it should be possible to observe this clash of defeasible concepts when a therapist encounters a family in treatment. There ought to be a pull on the therapist who meets a family system with a high degree of "pathology" (difference from the system from which the therapist comes) to behave in accordance with the family's system. Indeed, some conceptions of therapy

state that it is the therapist's job to offer the patient a new kind
of emotional experience, which could be translated in these terms
to "exerting a pull on the patient to join the therapist's frame of
reference, his labeling system, and not the converse." It is in this
situation of a therapist and family interacting that we ought to
see certain types of behavior; one social system must attempt to
induct the other into its frame of reference.

As implied above, individuals and groups struggle to preserve
the particular frames of reference they are accustomed to, and in
this struggle they can often be observed trying to defeat frames of
reference that contradict theirs This is seen not only in the behavior of the therapist who is deliberately trying to alter the behavior of his patient, but also in the conduct of the patient who
is resisting change. Several investigators have presented examples
in the literature. Thus, the manner in which the family of the
schizophrenic and the hospital of the schizophrenic resemble each
other has been burlesqued by Haley (18, p. 134). He has written
that the family of the schizophrenic is characterized by "a kind of
formless, bizarre despair overlaid with a veneer of glossy hope
and good intentions concealing a power-struggle-to-the-death
coated with a quality of continual confusion." Several pages later
in the same article, Haley uses precisely this phrase to describe
"the average mental hospital." Block (19) describes a phenomenon he refers to as "psychosocial replication" at a treatment center where patients reproduced their family systems in the milieu
of the institution. This can also be seen at institutions which do
not reproduce systems of the patients, but rather act counter-
phobically. For example, rehabilitation centers are known for
their cheery optimism and friendliness while the disabled population they are meant to serve clearly experiences rage and frustration. Other institutions like Alcoholics Anonymous reproduce the
alcoholic social system but remove one item: the alcohol. From
the foregoing examples it can be seen that the efforts of the individual or group to protect his own frame of reference for the interpretation of behavior commonly take the form of trying to induct dissident viewpoints into his own system, thus defeating the
opposition and demonstrating for us the defeasible nature of the
concepts here involved.

At the interfaces of different systems one can observe certain
characteristic dynamics. The first of these I call a *cycle*, where the

participants find themselves endlessly repeating the same things. For instance, at a lecture a questioner from the audience and the author, who was speaking, engaged in certain behavior. Aware of the possibility of cycles, the author asked his questioner how many times she thought the two of them had repeated themselves. Her guess was five times. We then sought to identify the aspects of our respective interpretive systems that conflicted. It turned out that the author had just described a family system similar to her own family of orientation, with a completely different interpretation than she would have given it. An understanding of the results of different frames of references, defeasible concepts, and use of the diplomatic "You may be right" ended the cycling.

Most people are also aware of *spirals* in which the repetition becomes increasingly intense; each interaction heightens the intensity even if just the opposite is intended. A rage is such a spiral, as is an anxious confusion. It is amazing to speak to participants afterwards because they are always overwhelmed by the obvious solution: if every action increases the spiral, do nothing. For instance, a child-care worker tried to break up a fight between two boys, succeeded in separating them, but then got into a spiraling rage reaction with one. The fight he was trying to break up was over, however; why he did not walk away? [1] In the end he had to stop the spiral by holding the child still with the aid of another assistant.

In order to demonstrate the defeasible nature of affects, I shall turn to a recorded and published transcription of a family interview. Lennard (20) and his co-workers have been particularly interested in "the family as a socialization system concerned . . . with enabling the child to identify and articulate *inner states*" [italics mine]. Although he begins with a typical notion of Whorf's binomial theorem variety (that there is a container and feelings inside it), Lennard also noted: "We are concerned with how parents elicit and pattern motives and feelings on the part of the child. Of particular importance here are the frequency and character of communications in which the parent interprets the child's experience, motives and feelings" (20). Reporting a series of dialogues, he noted that "the mothers shifted

1. The answer to this question is that he was attempting to induct the child into his interpretive system, in which such fights did not show "heart" (a delinquent value) but "mental illness" (also a value).

to this kind of [interpretive] communication" and observed "persistent efforts of the patient to change to another kind" (20);
such dialogues sound very much as though defeasible concepts
were being argued. In the following typical excerpt of a mother
and child, the mother is interpreting for her son and the choice
of affect label is being fought over.

Mother: What do you call it, er, er, ant . . . not antagonism,
          that's not the word. What is that other word? Um,
          still, there's a hostility underneath occasionally.
Patient: Shakiness, like, er. . . .
Mother: Maybe a little hostility towards me sometimes which
          crops up. Er. . . .
Patient: Do you have to use hostility?
Mother: A little, er, bitterness maybe
Patient: Yeah, that's
Mother: A little
Patient: That's better, or, or
Mother: A little
Patient: I, I think bitterness
Mother: Bitterness?
Patient: Yeah, er, the bitterness is something which I create
          myself
Mother: Yes
Patient: And you, and, and, er, I know it (20)

It seems to me entirely true, from this limited bit of dialogue,
that the patient does create his "bitterness" while the mother is
more inclined to prefer "antagonism" or "hostility," but it is still
a term offered by her.

Lennard reported that the mothers of schizophrenic children
whom he studied made more than twice as many comments about
how their husbands or sons were feeling than did control mothers. He assumed that these mothers were intervening too much
and too actively in comparison to control families. From the
point of view of affects as defeasible components of systems, it is
entirely possible that in the control families, fewer such statements are made because the remarks of the family members represent a shared frame of reference for interpreting behavior and
are more active in an interpersonal sense, while in the families of
schizophrenics we are watching an ongoing struggle.

Lennard tentatively concluded at the time of his study that

"the failure to relinquish symbolic control over the child's inner processes is characteristic of schizophrenic families" (20). It was the persistent notion that feelings are "inside" or imponderables that led him to a conclusion unlike the ones I have drawn. It is my contention that the family interactions he reported did not represent engulfing and intrusive activity on the part of the schizophrenogenic mother often cited in the literature; rather, these were extremely inefficient and crude efforts by the mother to have the family reach a consensus regarding the interpretation of behavior. Families and other social groups can be classified in terms of the efficiency shown in the rendering of "affect" judgments, by the degree of unanimity, and so forth. It would seem that the families of schizophrenic children represent extreme cases of conflict in frames of reference toward interpreting behavior. We might also ask who is opposing the so-called engulfing mother? Why hasn't she engulfed already? This raises the possibility of a struggle in the family for interpretive power, hitherto not seen. The question cannot be answered without further research; it is posed here only to demonstrate that the point of view I am espousing has certain heuristic consequences.

AFFECT AS TRANSACTION

"Do I cry because I'm sad or am I sad because I cry?" is a question in the James-Lange tradition that attempts to handle the problem of the relation between affect and behavior. It may now be seen as a category mistake. Crying (the behavior) and sadness (the affect label) are not in the same *category*, and no matter in what order they are put, one cannot be said to interact billiard-ball fashion with the other. My crying, as we have seen above, may be labeled by my social group as sadness, joy, effeminacy, rage, frustration, manipulation, or mental illness. It may be seen as involuntary autonomic nervous sytem activity, or it may be ignored. In any case, the label is in a different class from the behavior; it is in the class of judgments about behavior. Such judgments are, of course, themselves behavior. The choice of label may be made easily or only after considerable haggling, but in the view espoused here, it cannot be said to cause the crying in a linear sense of causality or vice versa. Parenthetically it may be noted that such disagreements regarding labels frequently lead to the diagnosis of "mental illness," as I have tried to show elsewhere concerning the label, "hysterical conversion reaction" (21).

If the approach presented here leads me to discard the James-Lange categorizing of affect and behavior, and to consider them different levels of the same transaction, it behooves me to make some statement about causality and the relationship between label and behavior. I must first distinguish between behavior that is possible but prohibited for a given individual to perform (such as crying), and behavior which is not in all behavioral repertoires. Each must be discussed separately.

In the first type of situation a group (or family), as a rule-governed system, may refuse to license the behavior in question ("men don't cry"). Although it is possible to break the rule, there are certain punishments inherent in so doing—essentially falling under the heading of desocialization. If, on the other hand, a family therapist is able to change the rules, the "new" behavior may show itself, producing an opportunity for an affect label. This is, of course, an oversimplification. The rule, "men don't cry," is frequently associated with an affect label of negative value ("crying is a womanly feeling") and change in rules offers an opportunity for a change in labels (crying is "sadness" and not "effeminacy"). The relationship between the label and the rule is reciprocal: as one changes so does the other. There is a complex circular causality. The therapist changes rules and labels as he works. The regulation, "men don't cry" and the label, "crying is a feminine feeling," essentially express the same rule and determine each other.

In the second case, where behavior is not restricted by rules but is absent from the behavioral repertoire, a somewhat different situation prevails. An abbreviated example will be used to show this. A boy of twelve and his rather young, lower-class mother find themselves in considerable difficulty: when they interact in a close fashion, for instance when the family therapist asks mother and child to sit together on a couch, there is a lot of behavior usually labelled embarrassment but which has underlying it considerable sexual tension. The mother indicates that she sees her son as "another man," and with men she has the limited behavioral responses of "fighting" or "making love." She is told by the therapist, "You have to learn to sit next to your son and do things in such a way that he doesn't get embarrassed and you don't feel you're dealing with another man." When and if this additional behavioral possibility is achieved, a label is sought for it: motherly love, affection, or whatever. With the emergence of the new behavior comes an opportunity for a new "affect."

In this view it becomes less important whether or not a label, commentary, or kind of behavior is to be called "an affect." Whether crying, for example, is to be called feminine or a woman's *feeling* becomes an issue more of phraseology than of anything else.

IMPLICATIONS FOR TREATMENT

Bringing together what has already been briefly touched upon with regard to treatment, there are three main areas for consideration:

1. The relativity of affect. Mead has said that the self is the reflected appraisal of others. Affects, in this view, are a special case of Mead's theorem. If the therapist can establish himself as the holder of interpretive powers, he can control behavior by the value judgments (the reflected appraisals in terms of affect and other labels) he assigns to such behavior. The dialogue between two psychiatrists, "You're feeling fine; how am I?" makes fun of this ability of psychiatrists to tell others what they are feeling.

2. System suction. A family, however, protects itself from such relabeling by attempting to induct outsiders into its system. The therapist can succeed in altering this system only if he resists such efforts. If we consider the example of mother and son cited above, it may be noted that therapeutic success might hinge on the male therapist's success in avoiding a pull or suction to deal with this woman on the terms she offers. To the extent that he can avoid the syndrome and model a different behavioral possibility, he will be able to offer the family a "new emotional experience." The success of therapy in other families can be related to the therapist's refusal to accept the family's labels for its different members. That is, he does *not* see certain members as inevitably psy-

chotic, or vicious, or heroic rescuers, etc., as they have been cast by the rest of their family.

The characteristics of a given social system are reasonably evident when all its members are seen together, as in the case of family therapy. It is also present, though less visible, in individual treatment, where the patient is seen as a representative of a system. Finally, the therapist, too, is part of a system. If we thus expand our frame of reference to consider the presence of two systems in the therapeutic situation, that of the family and that of the therapist, we can anticipate an inevitable conflict between them. The stated purpose of therapy is to alter in some way the behavior of the patient, and this entails alteration of the system to which he belongs. Changing any social system occurs through its confrontation by another system; in the case of therapy it is the therapist's, be it his own family system or a professional system with which he is in contact.

In order to resist the suction of the patient's system, therapists often lean on their association with other therapists. Many journal articles seem to consist of efforts of lonely men to keep in touch with a therapist system. Thus, we have the editorial comment of a new journal for therapists: " 'Any sincere therapist should be in continuous therapy for himself during his entire professional life!' This familiar comment expresses the awareness of a personal need for encouragement. So often the therapist feels drained. . . . We therapists find nurture for ourselves in the bosom of the family, and in encounters with colleagues" (22). This therapist-therapist dialogue, often disguised in obscure shoptalk, serves to insulate the therapist from the competitive systems he faces. Because circumstances require extreme allegiance at times of severe suction from other systems, the therapist systems tend to be narrow and cohesive. This can interfere with allegiance to larger groups, leaving psychiatry with numerous schisms having little to do with underlying theoretical differences.

3. Changing family rules. As I have suggested, the family may be seen as a rule-governed system. To the extent that family rules can be changed, certain behavior becomes available for commentary. As seen in the previous chapter, it is quite often necessary to obtain "releases" from ruling family members to obtain certain data and to enable certain behavioral operations to occur.

DISCUSSION

The process of ascribing a label to behavior subsequently called an affect is seen as an integral part of the behavior itself. The choice of label is a function of the observer's frame of reference for the interpretation of behavior and thus can vary between and within social groups. Affective labels represent both the behavior in question and the observer's interpretation of it; as such they are largely meaningful seen in the contexts of transactions between people rather than as inner states of one person. If affects are to be seen inside people, they must be amenable to change only by internal factors. Alternatively, affects seen as social processes may be influenced by other social processes. As our field develops, we may be able to paraphrase Maxwell and remark that psychological science is entering on the next stage of progress—that in which affects are no longer conceived of in terms of imponderables but in which the tensions and emotions of family and other natural groups are seen as determined by the configuration and motion of their systems.

CHAPTER FOUR

Topography: Is the Unconscious Necessary?

But a neurosis never says foolish things, any more than a dream.

SIGMUND FREUD

The title of this chapter is deemed by many psychiatrists to be an unthinkable question. Still others assume it to be a problem of interest to only psychoanalysts and perhaps philosophers. Yet when a psychiatrist whose orientation is predominantly organic attempts to explain hallucinations, or when a social psychiatrist tries to distinguish between mental health education and psychotherapy, each may find himself tending to conceptualize his problem by utilizing certain notions that have come to be called the concept of the unconscious, even if he does not subscribe to a psychoanalytic solution to these problems.

The purpose of this chapter is to show how this widespread concept can obscure and limit inquiry. I shall explore the possibility, first suggested by the American pragmatist Charles Sanders Peirce, that errors, mistakes, poor judgment, ignorance, or what he called *fallibility* can account for those phenomena explained in psychiatric theory by the concept of unconscious motivation.

THE SOURCE OF IGNORANCE

It is Descartes who, because he expressed himself so clearly, is held responsible for our current common-sense notions of how we think about things. On the surface the ideas he expressed seem perfectly reasonable; there are some thoughts and percepts which are intuitively obvious, which we just know, and other knowledge which is derived from these original building blocks. The argument is, however, usually reversed. That we derive our thoughts from previous thoughts seems unquestionable. Then logically there must be some irreducibly obvious first principles at the start of all this. The basic idea is as old as Plato, who described Socrates proving the intuitively evident character of geometry by merely asking questions of a slave—a process of delivering the obvious that Socrates is said to have likened to midwifery. Yet the Euclidian concept of space is no longer seen as intuitively obvious "in the clear light of reason," to use Descartes' metaphor. Looking back from the many geometries of the twentieth century and the space-time of Einstein, we now somehow doubt that we would have delivered the same baby that Socrates did.[1]

The problems discussed in this chapter arise from this assumption that there is intuitive knowledge. Although delivered by philosophers, the baby has been laid at psychiatry's door. Namely, there has always been a group of people who fail to have the most widely agreed upon obvious and intuitive thoughts and perceptions; they see things that aren't there, distort reality, and con-

1. For Descartes' philosophy, particularly his notion of intuition, see his "Sixth Meditation (1641)" in *Meditationes de Prima Philosophia* (1). Plato's use of intuition is to be found in the dialogue *Meno* (2). A reference to this dialogue and "midwifery" in relationship to the role of the therapist can be found in May (3). Peirce's doctrine of fallibility may be found in his *Collected Papers* (4) or, as reviewed in relationship to Descartes, in the chapter "The Assault on Cartesianism" in Gallie (5).

struct all sorts of peculiar beliefs. If there is intuitive knowledge, how are we to account for these madmen, for the source of this ignorance? What to do with them and how to explain these exceptions to the rule constitutes the history of psychiatry. The earliest and most obvious answer has been to assume that these mistakes —concerning things about which we cannot be mistaken—must be caused by damage to the brain, that the source of these errors is organic. There are, however, two other explanations: the concept of the unconscious, and that of fallibility (the doctrine that there is no intuitive knowledge).

THE ARGUMENT FOR THE UNCONSCIOUS

The concept of the unconscious was extensively propounded by Freud in papers intended for the general public. However, he also discussed the concept in his most technical and theoretical work. These writings have been the focus of a recent study by Holt. (6). Holt emphasizes that Freud's approach to a subject such as the unconscious was derived from the classical Greek tradition, a tradition that still existed among literate men of his times and whose methods, goals, and intentions differed from those of science.

The classical Greek tradition depended mainly on oral expression. Its medium was the spoken word. In this tradition the search for truth in most subject matter was undertaken by individuals whose only mode of communication was talking to each other. A commentary developed about how this dialogue should take place—what were its forms, how one was to do it best, and so forth. This methodology or criticism was called "rhetoric," the theory of persuasive spoken communication. At the time there was no science in the sense that we know it today, and no parallel commentary akin to rhetoric applied to it, which today we call the scientific method.

By examining Freud's manner of drawing conclusions in his entire corpus, and by carefully scrutinizing all Freud's arguments for the concept of a psychic unconscious in two of his major technical papers on the subject, Holt concludes that Freud rarely proved anything, in our modern, scientific sense of the word:

"The upshot of this survey of the means Freud used in what was ostensibly a search after truth is that he relied heavily on all the classical devices of rhetoric. The effect is . . . to persuade, using to some extent the devices of an essayist but even more those of an orator or advocate, who writes his brief and then argues the case with all the eloquence at his disposal" (6, p. 174).

It is, therefore, appropriate to treat the unconscious as non-scientific, as a basic assumption which cannot be proved or disproved but must be accepted as a given. In so doing, I am following Freud himself; in his *General Introduction*, among other places, he says he must be given this assumption or nothing satisfying can be made out of dreams and parapraxes (7, pp. 104–108). In a similar, more general argument Jones quotes Freud: "What speaks against the physiological conception is its unfruitfulness; for the psychoanalytic one it can be claimed that it has been able to make intelligible interpretation of thousands of dreams and has used them to achieve a knowledge of intimate mental life" (8. p. 215). Thus Freud's argument is not in the form of a scientific proof; his point is that such an assumption is practical in its consequences. It is also clear from this excerpt that Freud set his theory against organic ("physiologic") theory. In this formulation Freud argues not that dream interpretation leads to the unconscious, but the reverse—that the assumption of an unconscious leads to an interpretation of a dream. In modern terminology, Freud's argument is that the concept of an unconscious is a condition of the psychoanalytic game; if you are to interpret a dream you must grant this hypothesis. As such it cannot be tested but rather is a general *program* by which such activity is designed to proceed—a map, or a topography. In science as in psychoanalysis this fact is sometimes obscured and the converse is maintained: that such determinism is itself subject to proof (thus Freud could also maintain that dreams proved the unconscious). Such a reduction of this basic assumption or program to the status of a testable hypothesis leads to metaphysics, in this case the free will-determinism controversy, which I shall omit here.

Recent research has again brought to our attention the problem of evaluating the concept of the unconscious. Foulkes (9, p. 246) has reviewed the issue in dream research where discrepancies arise between psychoanalytic theory (that dreams stem from the unconscious) and electrophysiological studies:

No one who has had experience in collecting, examining or interpreting dreams can doubt that dreams often do express a person's
basic feelings and indicate his problems. And yet, the . . . data now
available suggest that we err in assuming that since this may be the
functional significance of the dream, the dream, therefore, must have
started with the expression of such feelings or the posing of such
problems. Rather it seems as if the dream allows the dreamer, eventually rather than immediately, to express himself in a rather profound way; it is not that the dream, by posing a basic challenge at its
outset, forces him to do this. . . . Dream theorists have tended to
assume . . . a necessary correspondence between interpretation theory and process theory . . . but this overlooks the possibility that
how a dream begins and what a dream becomes may be two entirely
different matters.

In a dream reported by Richard Jones (10, pp. 56–57), a female student dreams that she is looking for a job, walking all
over, until finally she locates one in which her employers seem
quite satisfied but which she herself finds grim—with an additional dream fragment in which her mother advises her to "get
out of that place" but she doesn't do so. In a commentary on the
dream, we are told that 1) in the wish-fulfillment analysis (that
is, in a transaction with a classical analyst), the emphasis would
be on streetwalking and prostitution fantasies; 2) the existential
interpretation would highlight the existential dilemma of finding
"oneself satisfied with" rather than being "satisfied with oneself";
3) the epigenetic analysis of Erikson would deal with initiative
(job-finding), industry (employers satisfied), autonomy (opposing mother), and so forth. If we add to these interpretations the
ones that might be produced from other schools of psychoanalysis, we see how entirely different is "what a dream becomes" in
a variety of situations within psychoanalysis; with different programs, one reaches different destinations, even when the differences are minor. A relationship based on Freud's rules, or any
one of the modifications mentioned above, can produce profundi-
ties of personal insight. As we shall see, a transaction obeying
radically different rules may lead in other directions.

THE ARGUMENT FOR FALLIBILITY

Up to this point, we have been discussing two complex ideas or philosophies. We have the point of view, usually ascribed to Descartes, that the truth will manifest itself unless one is organically impaired (insane)—and Freud's modification of it: that the truth will manifest itself unless there is unconscious resistance to it. Both would state, for instance, that the redness of a patch of paint is intuitively seen as red unless there is interference. The American pragmatist C. S. Peirce proposed a third alternative: that there is only one class of knowledge. He stated that no knowledge is direct or intuitively obvious, but that acts of judgment are involved even in perceptual experiences. He would assert the possibility of seeing the red patch as brown, just as he would endorse the possibility of being wrong about anything else. The notion that much of what we take for granted actually consists of judgments or inferences and is thus open to error led Peirce to call his theory "contrite fallibilism" (11). For Peirce, the perceptual "act" only *seems* different from other fallible judgments, such as those made in arithmetic.

Our feeling that perceptions are different from other judgments stems from our lack of awareness of the in-betweens, and from our assumption that there are special attributes of a real situation that distinguish it from a false or hallucinatory one. For example, if I add two and two and get five as the answer, and a few moments later correct my mistake, I still cannot change the fact that I *thought* two and two were five. Similarly, I cannot change the fact that I *saw* the colored patch as brown rather than red. Such errors need not be explained further for Peirce; one can only be contrite about them.

Recent cross-cultural studies seem to support this position. For example, in Navaho there is no distinction made between gray and blue; in Yoruba, no red-brown distinction. Linguistic patterns seem to determine a lot of what we tend to consider intuitive knowledge.

The argument for fallibility can be illustrated by a consideration of the use of the term *hallucination* and its relationship to dreams, viewed in a non-Cartesian framework. Recent findings in the area of dream research have strongly suggested that a dream is not known to be a dream intuitively, as the Cartesian view would advocate, but is identified as such only upon awakening (12). The experience is thought about and the judgment, "I have had a dream," is made. By implication, this Peirce-like point of view must also hold that one may err in this judgment and decide, "That was a real experience." It is possible to extend this argument to include dreamlike states that occur during the day. The judgment, "This is a night-dream," is similar in form to the judgment, "This is a daydream." In both situations a person may err.

As an illustration we may consider the case in which a young girl one day gives a firsthand report that her friend's sister had all her hair burnt off while bending over a fire. She tells several people about the accident, until later that day she begins to think about it and suspects that it might have been a dream. When she makes a telephone call to check, she is given information which shows that it was, in fact, a dream. She accepts this revised interpretation quite calmly and tells her friends that she was mistaken, that she had had a dream. They in turn report to her similar experiences they have had. None of those involved regard the situation as anything other than a mistake in judgment.

It is easy, however, to see how this experience could be labeled as hallucinatory. Only two further steps would be necessary to create a full-blown hallucination. First, the subject must see the occurrence as a new experience for her rather than related to common occurrences (failures in judgment). Secondly, the public must corroborate this; as Hawthorne put it in *The House of Seven Gables*, "the sick in mind . . . are rendered more darkly and hopelessly so by the manifold reflection of their disease, mirrored back from all quarters in the deportment of those about them; they are compelled to inhale the poison of their own breath, in infinite repetition" (13).

To summarize the foregoing discussion, the use of the term *hallucination* depends upon the theory of knowledge to which one subscribes. This theory of knowledge determines the subsequent careers of those involved and, in fact, is a program by which people guide their conduct, their transactions, and their very lives. Descartes' position, adopted by the organic school of thought, is that in some areas failures in judgments are not possible without an organic explanation. Freud's modification of this point of view is that a more profitable explanation is reached by employing the concept of the unconscious. Peirce's position attacks the fundamental assumption of both: that there are things about which we cannot be mistaken. If we turn to a discussion of errors and their relationship to the unconscious, it is possible to further differentiate these three points of view.

PARAPRAXES, ERRORS, AND IGNORANCE

In psychoanalysis, the functional significance of an error is to reveal a wish. But that does not have to mean that the error started with such a wish. As was seen above with respect to dreams, functional relationships do not necessarily require causal relationships. What a mistake becomes and what it began as may be two different things. Popper (14) has criticized in detail the point of view inherent in psychoanalysis which states that an error is the presence of something, constructed for the benefit of unconscious agencies of the mind which are not interested in, and in fact conspire to prevent, the truth from manifesting itself. This notion inevitably leads to the conclusion that once reality is unveiled, resistance analyzed, we have the power to be aware of it with insight, "to distinguish it from falsehood, and to know that it *is* truth . . . a most optimistic view" (14, p. 43). As Nietzsche put the ultimate expression of this view, "Every extension of knowledge arises from making conscious the unconscious" (15). Reducing it to absurdity, this view seems to hold that one would know Chinese if resistance to it were removed by psychoanalysis.[2] Obviously, this is not the contention of the analyst, but methodological confusion brings us to this point; it is sometimes forgotten that the Cartesian view posits two types of knowledge, direct and indirect. Nietzsche's statement overstates the Cartesian position and implies that all knowledge is direct and would be available if

2. As Dewey, another pragmatist, has pointed out, it is equally absurd to assume one would know Chinese if one were lectured (given "insight") about it. This has led to a search for other theories of instruction (16).

there were not unconscious resistance.

The doctrine of resistance is the psychoanalytic bulwark to the notion that the truth will manifest itself, once unveiled. External reality as well as the reality of psychoanalytic formulations are said to be recognized as "truth" when the conspiracies against them are removed. Reality testing goes on properly, this view maintains, unless there is "resistance" or "defense." As we have seen, Plato's Socrates in the *Meno* was able to help an uneducated slave "remember" the proof of a special case of a Pythagorean theorem. Similarly, the analyst incorrectly conceives of his job as helping the patient to see the light of psychoanalytic truths which, once unveiled or revealed, are intuitively obvious. Once again, it is helpful to distinguish between rhetoric, a persuasive technique, and a clear and distinct theoretical position. No one likes to consider himself ignorant and inept. I believe that patients themselves would often prefer to think of themselves as, for instance, castrating females and latent homosexuals rather than as simply embarrassingly inept and inexperienced with the opposite sex. We must be careful that a concept such as the unconscious, which started out as an interesting program for psychological investigation and manipulation, not become an excuse for incompetence. Kazin (17) has seriously discussed this problem with respect to creative writing. The notion that every sexual deviate is a poet *manqué*, he warns, is a wonderful opportunity for the "hack and the quack" to get together.

As an alternative to the foregoing, it would seem profitable to adopt Peirce's "fallibilism" and search for ignorance and cognitive deficits, seeking to correct them in therapy (whatever the rhetorical devices used). An educational model may be followed, as Sullivan was wont to do, instead of theoretically confining oneself to a discussion of defenses, the conspiracy against reality testing, underlying conflict, negative self-image, and so forth. In this way a climate is created in which error and ignorance are acceptable, in contrast to the prevalent situation today where asking why someone made a mistake is resolved by the conclusion that unsavory motivation lay behind the error. Peirce would simply argue for a social system in which an openness to learning and repair of error are feasible. Similarly, Sullivan said, "No essential difference exists between better integration of a personality to be achieved by way of psychoanalytic personality study and better integration to be achieved by an enlightened teacher of physics in demonstrating to his students the property of matter" (18). In this statement, Sullivan is clearly treating both experiences as educational. It is apparent that the properties of matter referred to above are not in the students' unconscious—that no amount of analysis will reveal them to the natural light of reason or to insight.

RELEVANCE TO PSYCHOTHERAPY

The three points of view I have been discussing can be illustrated by case material. In the first case, a young woman in therapy complains that she must achieve an orgasm by employing a spanking fantasy, most intense when she imagines her mother is spanking her. At this point the therapist has at least three options available to him. He may assume that such material is determined by the unconscious, that orgasms occur naturally unless there is some resistance. He may assume, although it is unlikely today, that orgasms occur naturally except in the case of local or organic mental disease. He may assume that orgasms are capable of being modified by error (Peirce's contrite fallibilism). Each of these positions has inherent in it a plan of action. In this case the patient was able to have an orgasm and drop the spanking fantasy (of many years' duration) in the course of a week when she discovered that if she waited, she could have an orgasm without the fantasy. Since then (one year), the problem has not recurred. This problem, which certainly seems to resemble that which psychoanalytic theory is designed to handle, could also be dealt with in terms of ignorance of the cognitive map of sexual stimulation.

The second case concerns a patient who had difficulty falling asleep and entered therapy asking specifically, "What is preventing me from getting to sleep?" When asked what she meant, she indicated, in a manner that Popper would enjoy, that there must be some mysterious agent preventing her from sleeping. Here again the problem—in this case sleep onset—can be approached from an educational vantage point. The therapist has the option of saying that ignorance of sleep onset techniques is responsible for the patient's inability to sleep, or, alternatively, that sleep is a natural state which is achieved if there is no resistance involved, such as fear of death or dreaming. The third possibility would be that of an organic basis for sleep disturbance.

An interesting clinical sidelight on the concept of fallibility is the notion that various symptom complexes might be performed with more or less skill. It is commonly assumed that a psychiatric entity—for instance, paranoid behavior—is effectively executed by all who display it rather than that standards of competence can be applied here also. As a corollary it is usually believed that all paranoid symptoms have maximum and infallible benefit to those involved rather than that the greater portion of such behavior, like that of most behavior, is merely adequate. For example, while paranoid behavior is often poorly carried out, a competent paranoid can create a hostile environment in perfect keeping with his subjective expectations; in the superbly performed paranoid maneuver the others who are involved can be made to display foolishness, or enraged and even deranged behavior. This stabilizes the life of the initiator in the sense of supplying him with a clear and present problem apparently originating with his misguided friends, relatives, or acquaintances. It also delays recognition of his pathology by himself and others.

THE HEALING POWERS OF EDUCATION

The distinction usually drawn between education and psychotherapy is largely based on the concept of the unconscious and the general family of concepts involving an inner mental life. Psychotherapy is said to change the unconscious and education to add to the conscious. Even within a psychoanalytic context this distinction has been challenged, as in the observation by Sanford that "there is a common notion that changes so profound as to involve the relations of id, superego and ego can be brought about . . . only by means as thoroughgoing as psychoanalysis or deep psychotherapy. I'm suggesting that changes of a pretty fundamental kind can be brought about by regular education procedures . . ." (19). If the basic assumption of the unconscious is questioned, as I suggest, then both education and psychotherapy must be completely redefined according to other criteria, and the validity of the distinction traditionally made between them must be reevaluated.

From the point of view of social psychiatry, psychotherapy is seen as using the tutorial method (in individual psychotherapy), the seminar method (in group therapy), and the classroom method (in mental hygiene education). The superiority of the tutorial method in most cases should not be allowed to obscure the basic similarities of these situations in terms of program and intentions. Of course, the subject matter, the psychotherapeutic curriculum, is considerably different in terms of its *manifest content* than the school curriculum, but closer scrutiny reveals their formal similarities. The format and agenda are more often disguised in an educational setting and made explicit in psychotherapy, and this contributes to the seemingly great differences between the two situations.

Like Peirce, Vygotsky (20) has asserted that we are not necessarily aware of exercising judgments in certain contexts. He claimed that the concepts learned by a child can be divided into spontaneous concepts (e.g., "brother") which are not initially regarded as concepts by the child although he uses them correctly, and non-spontaneous concepts (e.g., "exploitation") which are actively and deliberately taught. The child's awareness that "exploitation" is a concept and can be managed as such occurs before he realizes this with regard to "brother." Within the context of the foregoing discussion, perceptions can be seen as special varieties of spontaneous concepts.

Vygotsky proceeded to observe that awareness of spontaneous concepts can be taught. This notion, that children's awareness of judgmental processes works downward to spontaneous concepts, becomes identical with the process of the analysis of the unconscious ego in psychoanalytic terminology. This has been said another way in the literature of existential psychotherapy. Here the non-neurotic is defined as one who is not imprisoned by automatic perceptual judgments; he is acutely and sometimes painfully aware that he actively chooses his reality in an absurd world. Camus, for instance, presents the difficult and extreme case that Sisyphus must actually be regarded as happy in spite of his perpetual torture precisely because he is aware of his situation and free to choose his emotion, that he is not bound to perceive his condition "spontaneously." In the same vein, Bettleheim writes of concentration camp conditions and speaks of an inner freedom to choose one's attitude toward one's destiny, no matter how bleak it may be.

Existential case illustrations describing active awareness of usually automatic judgmental processes cloud the general issue because they so often apply only to the extreme situation. By describing virtuoso performances of extraordinary adaptation, they do not seem relevant to everyday life. But to relieve ordinary distress, the task of the therapist is to convince the patient to accept responsibility for his perceptions and, in Vygotsky's terms, other spontaneous concepts. This eventually leads to attempts to consensually validate what were previously uncritically held assumptions and beliefs. Thus a basic principle of psychotherapy is the importance of identifying and correcting imprisoning judgments that may create inaccurate perceptions of self and reality. Such judgments are assumed in most cases to be either spontaneous, unconscious, or acquired in childhood. Psychotherapy is in this sense given the assignment of remedial education, not for what was omitted at school but for what has not been taught correctly at home.

By the same token, social psychiatrists can accept the assignment of examining the school curriculum. If we reject the usual dichotomy between psychotherapy and education, then the school must also be seen as teaching, perhaps unwittingly, rules of behavior and social competence which sometimes may even conflict with academic goals. Analysis of an ordinary classroom scene may serve as an example. In a first-grade class I once observed, the children were supposed to be having fun by playing games; in this case the game was singing. The teacher had made up rather dull music and verses in which she could substitute words, written on large cards, in order to carry out her hidden agenda, which was learning to read. Further observation revealed a hidden subagenda: how to behave in class. Whether or not a child knew the answer (could play the game of singing by reading the word on the sign) was not as important as decorum: raising his hand, waiting to be called on, sitting quietly, and so forth. In short, while the teacher's apparent concern was reading instruction, it became apparent that more was going on: teaching decorum had the highest priority. In this context it is noteworthy that many effective teachers in lower-class schools achieve their results by merely omitting this particular hidden subagenda and permitting behavior which seems noisy and disorganized according to middle-class standards. Analysis of classroom events along the lines of this illustration is in some ways comparable to anthropological field studies. Thus when Jules Henry (21), an anthropologist, observed an urban classroom, he found as much to study as when he had investigated the behavior of primitive American Indians. Accordingly, to the extent that the social psychiatrist can be helpful in studying this level of the educational curriculum, one is tempted to say that education is too important to be left to the professional educator.

DISCUSSION

Freud's concept of the unconscious is seen as a basic assumption supported by certain rhetorical devices in his writings and in therapy itself, which allows certain transactions to take place which the patient enters into with the expectation that he will benefit from them. He is inducted into a relationship with the analyst where certain rules are followed (whereby the analyst has definite advantages and delegated powers). Here it is important only to emphasize that the concept of the unconscious and the analyst's interpretative powers may be used as effective devices for personality study and change, but such a notion does not imply that the unconscious has been or could be "proved" by scientific method, or that all adaptive problems are to be attributed to it.

Freud's concept of the unconscious is seen as an important modification of what today is called a Cartesian theory of knowledge. It takes the position, in essence, that adaptation (mental health) and acceptance of the "truth" of psychoanalytic exegesis is something about which one does not err unless some disruption (what Popper calls a conspiracy and Freud a resistance) occurs. Methodologically this position would state that the madder an action, the more can be gained by making it "rational" (finding the resistance or unconscious forces that make it happen). The important point is that the Cartesian criterion of madness—that about certain things we are never mistaken—is accepted.

The psychoanalyst makes two related claims. First, the behavior he deals with falls within Descartes' category of direct, infallible knowledge—that which is not learned but which is intuitively obvious. Second, failures in this direct knowledge cannot actually be failures at all but are intended by an unconscious agency of the mind. They are, in fact, highly complex, successful unconscious modes of behavior which preclude the need to claim that the individual is organically ill. For example, if I fail to get a job as an actor, I can say that I failed to do something I am intuitively capable of doing and my failure actually reflects the success of my unconscious. I, therefore, need a psychoanalyst, not an acting teacher. There are some, like Kazin, who take exception to the wide range of problems considered intuitive knowledge and would regard acting, in the above example, as classified incorrectly. However, in the situation where I see something that is not there, the notion of the unconscious is quickly evoked and similar reasoning is employed. Peirce, on the other hand, with his concept of contrite fallibilism, challenges the very criterion of madness accepted by Descartes and Freud. His point is that no knowledge, adaptive behavior, or even perception is direct and intuitive. Because it is not taught in school does not mean that it is not learned behavior and, therefore, open to error. This point has been illustrated by considering so-called hallucinations that result from incorrectly judging whether something is a dream or daydream. What characterizes a hallucination is not failure of intuitive knowledge but failure in the correction of error. That in relatively rare instances such individuals are deemed mentally ill is a function of two things: their social undesirability and the community's intolerance of error by its failure to encourage repair.

The behavioral scientist or practitioner who is confined to a doctrine that obscures the fundamental role of knowledge and its absence, who cannot ask the question asked in the title of this chapter, is limited in his capacity for inquiry. Any doctrine, whether physical or psychological in approach, that does not consider the consequences of ignorance detracts from personal responsibility for learning and teaching and the fundamentally moral nature of the problem with which we are continually faced: to learn to learn—even in those areas like perception and social competence that have always been considered intuitive.

CHAPTER FIVE

The Shape
of Time:
Epigenetics

It was toward springtime, . . . and the teacher
said: "I saw something the other day and I wonder
if any of you have seen it? If you know it, don't
say what it is. I went out and I saw coming up
from the ground something about 10 inches high
and on top of it was a little round ball of fluff,
and if you went woof, a whole galaxy of stars flew
out.

"Now, what was it like before the little ball of
stars appeared?" the teacher asked. One fellow said
it was a little yellow flower, like a sunflower, only
very small.

"And what was it like before that?"
A little girl said it was like a little green umbrella,
half closed, with a yellow lining showing out.

"Yes, but what was it like before that?" One of
them said it was a little rosette of green leaves
coming out of the ground.

"Now, do you all know what it is?" the teacher
asked. They were ready to explode. They roared
back, DANDELION!

"And did you ever pick dandelions?" Most of them

said yes, but he said, "No. You can't pick a dandelion. That's impossible. Bill, what did you get—
some of those balls of fluff? And you didn't get any
rosette of leaves—all you got was a ball of white
fluff?

"A dandelion is all of this, so whatever you
picked, you only got a fragment of something or
other. You can't pick a dandelion, because a dandelion isn't a thing; it's a performance. And you
know, every living thing is a performance, even
you.

. . . "The big thing is not to ask, 'What's this,' but
to ask, 'What's going on here?' "

ARTHUR A. MOOR (1)

GROWTH, DEVELOPMENT, AND STRUCTURE

The dandelion is that segment of the performance, the process,
which lasts, which slows down to such a snail's pace that we see it
as a thing, a form. The slowness of its evolving pattern serves to
dissect process into structural units. In some ways it is the opposite of motion pictures where, past a critical flicker fusion frequency, the structural images—in this case photographs—com-
bine into a performance. Time-lapse photography creates a similar effect, and would convince us that "dandelion" is indeed the
name of a performance rather than an object.

Distinctions such as "structure," "movement," and "developmental process" are not out there in the external world but relate
to the critical fusion frequency of the observing system (eye or
camera). Such definitions are determined by characteristics of the
observer as well as the observed. For example, if I am on a train
and there is a book in my compartment, to me the book is sta-
tionary. But from another vantage point, standing on the ground
beside the moving train, the book is speeding along. There is actually no absolute speed of the book, only a relative speed or
speed within a context. Just as the judgment of movement is a
function of the physical location of the observer, judgments
about structure and process depend on one's temporal vantage
point. If we think of a spectrum of phenomena that varies in du-

ration, those which are fast and short are typically regarded as processes while those which are slow and prolonged are seen as structures. Both are ranges within the same spectrum, though, consisting of similar events and varying predominantly in terms of speed and duration. All of these are contexts which inevitably include some sort of relationship or interaction between the observer and the observed. Therefore speed, motion, immobility, structure, and developmental process are relative to these considerations.

The task for social psychiatry is not the explanation of developmental process but the explanation of form or structure; not why there are events, but why they sometimes appear to freeze into things. We are concerned in social psychiatry with a theory that postulates process as its fundamental fact, and so this chapter precedes the one on structure. To clear out the undergrowth of pre-evolutionary genetic theory from psychiatry, it is necessary to realize that both Darwin and Lamarck made the same basic assumption: evolutionary process is basic and the forms or structures momentarily seen are secondary. This emphasis on process over structure is thus not a new idea; it is new only in the tradition of psychiatric thought. It can entail either relatively minor or extreme changes in the nature of our conceptualizations. The physicist Bridgeman provides an example of the latter in his discussion of the electron, something we habitually regard as a structure: " . . . the electron . . . paradoxically has no identity, so that we cannot follow a particular electron about in its adventures as we could a mote of dust suspended in the atmosphere. . . . An electron is an aspect of a total situation, the major part of which is the rest of the apparatus. We should not talk about 'electrons' as such, but rather say: 'Under such and such conditions the apparatus electrons' " (2, p. 176). Bridgeman presumably would include the observer as part of the total situation.

Genetics emerged as a subspeciality of biology in the preevolutionary period of science, before Darwin argued for the primacy of process over structure. As a result, early geneticists applied the reverse emphasis, relying on the simple premise that all genetics is growth of a given structure. They assumed that living things duplicate themselves as small replicas of the adult structures and these grow to adult size. In this view, an acorn is simply a folded-up tree. The most famous and, in retrospect, outlandish, example of this approach was made possible by the advent of the micro-scope. Scientists examined the human sperm and saw a perfect duplication of a human child with what seemed to be a nightcap on his head. This little homunculus, "discovered" by the micro-scope, was presumed to develop by growing larger and larger but changing in no other aspect. This general approach to genetics is called *preformistic*, emphasizing that what is, was. What is pre-formed is the homunculus or some other structure that grows. The Freudian theoretical position on genetics merely reverses the usual emphasis on adult form, saying instead that the tree is acorn-ish, rather than that the acorn is tree-ish. This leads to the conclusion that the adult psychologically is a grown-up child. In theory it does not really matter whether one insists that the acorn is a small oak or the oak a large acorn except as it supports a spe-cial argument in Freudian theory which will be discussed below. The fallacy, the preformistic error, is the same (unless one wishes to use "postformistic" for Freud's idea). As I have noted in pre-vious chapters, it is our observing system or language that often leads us to see a performance as an object, a process as a structure —to "objectify," in Whorf's terminology. One gathers from Whorf that a Hopi Indian would have no problem in avoiding a preformistic view, although one begins to suspect that we should give Whorf more credit and the Hopi language less for really grasping the nature of this problem.

The alternative to preformistic doctrine is called the *epigenetic* view. Epigenesis, or "development," in the sense that it is being used here, is merely a term that helps to express the distinction between process and structure, which, as noted earlier, are quite arbitrarily defined for us by the nature of our observing systems. Before dealing with the concept of epigenesis in detail, we must detour to explore a series of ideas about time, the frequent con-founding of spatial and temporal metaphors, the rise of the no-tion of metachronicity, and alternative models of time.

TWO-TENSE AND THREE-TENSE LANGUAGES

In addition to judgments about speed or duration in defining a phenomenon as either process or structure, our language and our concept of time also influence such definitions. In the English language we have three tenses: past, present, and future; and we rely primarily on spatial metaphors that require events to be assigned a physical location in space. Both of these qualities lend themselves to the description of structure but make it difficult to describe process. At best we can use spatial metaphors only to express temporal concepts, and often time and space become confounded in our formulations. As Whorf has pointed out, we say in English "ten days" as if it were an expression similar to "ten bottles," and "ten days is greater than nine days" as if it were like "ten bottles is greater than nine bottles." To be accurate, we should say "the tenth day is later than the ninth" (avoiding the plural "ten days" and the spatial metaphor "greater than.") Whorf has suggested that a language system such as Hopi that stresses temporal metaphors and has only two tenses, earlier and later, "would seem to correspond better to the feeling of duration, as it is experienced" (3, p. 143). Because of the predominance of spatial metaphors in Western languages, the concepts of inner space and historical time were invented to accommodate what was difficult to place in outer (or environmental) space. The extent to which our language is permeated with spatial metaphors is illustrated by Whorf: " . . . we can hardly refer to the simplest nonspatial situation without constant resort to physical metaphors. I 'grasp' the 'thread' of another's argument, but if its 'level' is 'over my head' my attention may 'wander' and 'lose touch' with the 'drift' of it, so that when he 'comes' to his 'point' we differ 'widely,' our 'views' being indeed so 'far apart' that the 'things' he says 'appear' 'much' too arbitrary, or even 'a lot' of nonsense!" (3, p. 146). The grammatical problem that challenges social psychiatry is thus to use the spatial metaphors and three tenses of English, since we have no choice unless we communicate in mathematics, and yet to describe without preformistic errors things that are intangible: the assumptions about genetics and about time.

THE HISTORY OF HISTORY

Like genetics, time can be considered in a preformistic framework. That is, we can think, as the early Greeks did, of a *preformed* fate. This idea of predestination was probably the first time model to be used in Western thought. Although past, present, and future tenses existed in the language, events were described in essentially a historical or nonchronological order. The *Iliad,* for example, consists of bits of narrative, like a series of snapshots arranged in some personal order and not like a motion picture epic. Homer's sense of time, compared to ours, was vague and irregular. The story of the *Iliad* starts in the tenth year of the Trojan War and concludes without even touching on the capture of Troy. The fact that the author plunges into his subject, which was in modern times a basis for literary praise, is not a sign of his genius. Actually, he starts at the beginning of his subject, and he says so quite plainly. He is composing a story about a quarrel between Achilles and Agamemnon. Slowly, the reader begins to realize that for Homer, *there is no such thing as chronological history.* Even this story about Achilles and Agamemnon, one hot-tempered and one prideful, could have been related in an orderly narrative fashion, but it isn't. Homer does not have our sense of time, and it is completely beyond him to write a "case history" of a quarrel any more than what we usually understand by a "history" of a war. It is a bit of a shock to discover that there is a history of history, or that there wasn't always a linear past, present, and future—a three-tense conceptual world.

The next model to be adopted evolved from the tripartite model of weaving. What have now become identified as past, present, and future in our formulation of events were for the Bronze Age Greeks three people, the three Fates, who wove patterns in cloth. The reason for having three Fates seems derived from the fact that weaving as a household task in Greece was commonly carried out by three different people. It is possible to think of other situations on which the ancient Greeks might have modeled their concept of time, or even other ways to break up the process of weaving. For instance, Onians (4) mentions a northern European notion of eight stages of weaving.

The process of weaving involved three people, each with a different task. It is noteworthy that we represent these three tasks incorrectly today. Everybody now thinks of the three Fates as spinning, weaving, and cutting the thread of life. Onians (4) has corrected this image by studying weaving in ancient Greece. He concluded that the first step was the weighing of the raw material, the next was spinning, and the final step was weaving it into a fabric. The first step, the weighing of the raw material, was meant to check on how much work was being done and was usually carried out by a trusted servant. The second step, spinning, involved holding the raw wool in the lap. The expression occasionally heard today, "It is in the lap of the gods" (in other words, it is up to fate), is a reference to this aspect of the weaving model. The *final* act is weaving, and not cutting the thread, as we would have it today. This difference between our conception and that of the Greeks is significant because it entails the extent of difference in our respective beliefs in a preformed fate. In early Greece the final act is seen as weaving because this indicates the finality of one's career in life at birth: one's fate is set with the completion of the cloth with its tribal (not individual) design, in which infants were swaddled. It is natural that we should distort this image to the finality of death (cutting the string) because, as we now believe, death is our only certain or preformed fate, and because death is much more significant in a society that emphasizes individuality.

In short, the notions of life then and now are completely different. Our "fate" is constantly being woven, and when it is done we die. In the Bronze Age, man's fate was woven at birth. Time, for the early Greek, was a binding to the immutable course of life. Fate as a concept actually served well to explain what happened to him. Although fate was eventually rejected in many situations as an approach to life, the three stages, past, present, and future, were incorporated into later, linear time models where events were conceptualized in historical sequence.

Intervention in the Greek fate model had to take place on Olympus, so to speak, since man, as we have discussed in Chapter Two, was not seen as the initiator of his own behavior. Apollo in some later myths is said to have made the fates drunk in order to save a friend, but there is even some question in mythology whether Zeus is not subject to them. Achilles says: "Don't you see me too, a fine big man. My father is a brave man, my mother is a goddess: yet I too have death and fate fast upon me. The day shall come, morning or evening or midday, when someone shall take my life too in battle . . ." (5, p. 246). The expression "fate fast upon me" meant that the design woven by the fates was figuratively worn or tied around him. Not only was weaving the model but it was extended to a clothing metaphor. We still think of "shedding an identity," "stripping ourselves bare," and so forth. The whole message of the *Iliad* to the effect that the gods have their way, that there is some larger pattern that cannot be seen, modified, or controlled, is challenged by our late Iron Age concepts. Therefore it has become necessary to invent a different time scheme—the historical.

The relationship between history as a time concept and individuality can best be expressed by the series of assertions: I, my inner space and content, do not change (even if my body does); I am unique, my essential individuality and identity are timeless. What happens is that I, the individual, travel over time just as I travel over space in a sequence of measured steps. It is as if I, my inner space and only my inner space, am on a train sitting quietly. Everything else changes. History is what passes by the window (and even my body is part of that history.) Thus if I do not change, if I am unique, or if I am to be considered a firm individual particle, the difference that one sees between me and others like me is a difference of position, of coordinates, of where I am and where they are, and how I got there, of the sequence, of where and how my train has taken me. (The political and social importance of the assertion of individuality has been discussed in previous chapters.)

With this background of the history of history it is possible to take a wider view of time models. Fate and history are only two of the possible shapes of time.

FOUR SHAPES OF TIME

There is a sharp dichotomy today between those psychotherapists who think that the analysis of antecedent events in a patient's life history must precede behavioral change and those therapists who believe that current behavior can most effectively change by focusing on what they call "the here and now." The latter practitioners go so far as to say that our cultural blind spot most responsible for mental illness is a lack of a sense of immediacy. A third position is that important change in behavior is not possible, that we all have our appointments in Samara. In fact, Freud can be seen as sharing this view in large measure—although many of his followers were almost utopian in their expectations of absolute cure through Freud's treatment methods. The major trajectory of our life, Freud thought, is set (in the lap of the gods). We can modify only minor aspects of life and resign ourselves to our "fate." Fate is expressed in Freud's thought in terms of the genetic factors of gender ("Anatomy is destiny"), strength of instincts, and constitutional endowments, together with the influence of past experiences and the insoluble conflicts between society and our individual passions. In fact, his notion of the timelessness of the unconscious and of the predetermined inevitability of infantile neurosis, and even the strategy of life he offered patients, are Greek.

A fourth view, which is held by some psychotherapists but more prominently by laboratories doing "anthropological" research in families and non-verbal behavior, proposes that an understanding of behavioral cycles in a patient's life, even the repetitions in a hour of observed family transactions, is of the utmost significance for psychotherapists interested in behavioral change.

We are therefore confronted with four prominent views of time. Forced as we are to use structural models, we can say that each point of view has a shape. The historical point of view sees events as following a line; the here-and-now position sees time as a point; the fatalists see time as some sort of unalterable design fixed forever, and those interested in repetition see time as a circle or spiral.

These four points of view can be presented more clearly through examples:

1. *Linear Time.* Any historical work offers an example of linear (straight-line) time. Thus Theodore Draper writes of understanding the Vietnam political negotiations: " . . . As each move and manoeuver comes into the news, it tends to live a life of its own, undefiled by previous moves and manoeuvers. Yet, as every historian knows, history is not made that way, and it is necessary to put the pieces together to understand any one of them. The fate . . . [of an incident] cannot be understood by itself, divorced from the events which led up to it or the consequences that flowed from it . . . " (6, p. 17).

2. *Time as a point.* In contrast to the historian's linear formulation, Zen Buddhists, Fromm, Buber, and those psychotherapists who frequently call themselves existentialists regard the point as

an important spatial model of time. Watts writes: "Zen is a liber-ation from time . . . it becomes obvious that there is no other time than this instant, and the past and the future are abstrac-tions without any concrete reality" (7, pp. 199–200). In this time concept it is "immediacy" that is clarifying.

3. *Time as a fixed pattern.* A more complex pattern is concep-tualized by those who concentrate on presumably fixed events, which they rhetorically refer to as "natural history." Perhaps the most striking example is the formulation that could be written "infancy, childhood, adolescence, adulthood, old age"—a natural history so thoroughly accepted that Aries' book *Centuries of Childhood* comes as a shock to us (8). In it, he carefully docu-ments a period when there was no socially identified period of childhood. Children were dressed in small-sized adult clothes and were drawn by artists as little men. Until the nineteenth century children were "deprived" of childhood as it is known and insisted on today; but at the same time, there were more child prodigies "Teenage" is an even more recent and perhaps less appreciated invention of this viewpoint. There was an era, not so long ago, when one was either a child or an adult.

4. *Time as Circular.* The basic issues in circular time are repe-tition (cycles) and accumulation (spirals). When time is con-ceived as a straight path through space, repetition tends to be ov-erlooked, and it is the unique element that stands out as notewor-thy. If, on the other hand, time is thought of as spiral-shaped, the converse becomes true. Among the Hopi, for example, the two-tense grammatical language structure and orientation leads to an appreciation of cyclic rather than single events; it is the repeated rather than the exceptional that is noticed. According to a linear time model, for example, each day represents a potential clean slate or fresh start. But for the Hopi, "It is as if the return of the day were felt as the return of the same person, a little older but with all the impresses of yesterday, not 'another day,' i.e., like an entirely different person" (3, p. 151). Hopi dance ceremonies with their endless repetition hour after hour express the apprecia-tion of and the importance attributed to repetition.

With this time model and language structure, the Hopi ana-lyzes the world in terms of events (or as Whorf prefers to call it, "eventing,") rather than in terms of structures and objects. One might assume that in Hopi the reverse of our problems occur: He can conceptualize with ease a world of process, but has trouble with growth and structure. He might have difficulty with keeping accounts and reporting sequential events in a historical framework, but has no trouble with the notion of structures as processes of long duration. Thus in Hopi one of the basic points of this chapter is being made all the time: the primacy and variety of process. We learn further from Hopi that repetition becomes more significant and noticeable under these conditions.

In the framework of cyclical time, if there must be sequence because of the structure of our language, the line is bent on itself. This maneuver does two things: first, it satisfies our language in its linear form, second, it gets around the problem by curving the line back on itself so that there is actually no sequence, since it is not clear where to start in a loop. Circular causality is no causality at all, but a way in Western language to describe simultaneously occurring events.

When repetition is emphasized, the past, present, and future in terms of the historical model are not distinct; they are merely different cycles of essentially the same process. There is no neatly placed series of structures along a tapemeasure called time, no brilliant structure majestically filling the present, as the Zen master would have it, and no preformed structure in which the Greeks felt trapped.

METACHRONICITY

There is, of course, no reason why any one theorist in psychiatry must use only one time model. Freud, for example, used several. His countertransference-transference notion is an expression of immediacy (all that we need to know is what is going on in the here-and-now). His oral-anal-phallic-genital notion relates to the time model of a natural history; the repetition compulsion, to the cylical model of time. As with all of Freud's writings, one can emphasize one aspect over the other, as I have done in the preceding discussion of preformistic theory. But, in general, he was capable of taking multiple points of view. Thus his notion of metapsychology, or the use of multiple models of an event, allowed him a particular kind of freedom, a kind of freedom which he took with his concept of time also, but about which he never commented. Perhaps he would have coined a term like *meta-chronicity,* as Gioscia (9) has done recently, in order to license the use of several time models.

There is a subtle but important reason for taking multiple points of view. As Sapir has said, "We see and hear and otherwise experience very largely as we do because the language habits of our community predispose certain choices of interpretation" (3, p. 132). Freud's genius consists of deliberately setting out to use several language habits. He was systematically (deliberately) unsystematic.

All explanations of complex processes use some model. For instance, time in the Western world uses some sort of visually perceived (spatial) model. In the Orient there are models of time taken from the burning of incense; that is, models based on smell instead of sight. Whatever the model, by emphasizing one aspect of the situation, it suppresses others. Whatever the advantages of using smell as the basis of a time concept, it must replace the advantages of sight. Therefore, whenever there is a forced choice between models, in this case models of time, to choose one is to lose three others. If all four models of time could be used in observing and explaining some event, much would be gained by these multiple fixes. It is nevertheless apparent that some models are better for certain things. As I have suggested, growth and structure are seen most clearly in historical or fatalistic time models.

Perhaps a specific application of the different time models to a single situation will illustrate the increased understanding that can be provided in this way. For example, a curious natural phenomenon is the extended predator-victim relationships of distinct animal groups, such as that between hyenas and wildebeests. When a hyena pack picks off newborn wildebeests on the plains of Africa one option is to focus upon the individuals involved. Under these circumstances, the hyena needs no introduction to us. He is the proverbial despicable coward who terrorizes the innocent and the weak. The mere sight of him arouses our dislike; his elimination is the strategy of choice. This conceptualization of events follows the linear or historical point of view.

From another approach, this encounter can be said to have, at least, the virtues of being genuine and authentic. As such, we can appreciate that "this is darkest Africa." Such a jarring juxtaposition of views is hard to assimilate or translate into human interaction, although this has been done in literature. Thus, Norman Mailer (10) has defended (infamously, it has been charged) the "authenticity" of the juvenile delinquent's act of smashing an old storekeeper over the head with a gun. More abstractly, Camus' (11) hero Meursault in *The Stranger*, has an iconoclast's view of the individualistic position, and does not construct events in sequence but simply considers the raw facts; although in the novel he is judged in court as a born criminal type, Camus indicates that the former orientation has the virtues of genuineness and authenticity. This, in short, represents the "time as a point" model.

From a third point of view, the hyena's career is to be a scavenger; the natural history of his species inevitably leads to such behavior. Finally, adopting the fourth or cyclical viewpoint, there is a sudden expansion of focus. The hyena and wildebeest disappear as structures, as individuals. What is noteworthy in this context is a series of processes and their repetitions. There exist two systems, the wildebeest herd and the hyena pack, which repeatedly impinge on one another in a very special way. It becomes evident that the hyena pack lives in harmony with other systems such as the bird flock or the jackal pack, which also live together with it and the wildebeest herd. On reflection it becomes apparent that the elimination of hyenas would eliminate the wildebeests: the herd would overgrow its food supply, its composition would tend toward old, feeble, sick animals, disease would spread, and so forth. For the wildlife manager, the question becomes how many wildebeests the hyenas should be allowed to kill in order to keep the herd's composition at given proportions or size, for what desired outcome. The hyena is actually drawn to the newborn wildebeest because there have been many wildebeests calving at the same time in this location, and the smell of placental blood attracts him. In rather far-fetched teleological terms, he is drawn by the potential population explosion and the danger to the wildebeest herd.

What starts out in the historical framework as a repellent situation involving the individual hyena and the newborn wildebeest becomes in this model a repetition, a cycle that has long endured. To save individual wildebeests may ultimately endanger the entire herd. This "ecological consciousness," as the conservationists call it, challenges much of Western political and religious philosophy.

EPIGENETICS

The term *epigenetics* is another example of a spatial metaphor that attempts to cope with an intangible. *Epi* means "on, against, upon." This prefix, unfortunately, is often taken in its literal sense, which suggests the placement of one structure upon another, as in the case of a pacemaker that governs the unfolding growth of another structure. However, *epi* can be used in a more figurative sense as a view of a totality from above, whereby *epi* represents the viewpoint of the observer. It is because of its more common spatial interpretation that epigenetics has been seen *incorrectly* as a preformed pattern with something superimposed *on* it, such as a pacemaker. Thus Jones writes: "The epigenetic view conceives of maturation as inexorably following an endogenously unfolding program with a pace-setting schedule of its own. This program [the maturational sequence of Freud's libido theory] is modulated and given ultimate substance by development of an interactional order" (12, p. 16). This approach still adheres to the "unfolding" idea of preformistic theory but combines it with a governor that regulates the pace. It is this governor that apparently is presumed to have some interaction with the environment.

In the nineteenth century the theory of epigenetics did include the assumption of a *nisus formativus,* a formative agent that produced the ovum out of an undifferentiated mass. Comparing the little homunculus inside the sperm, with his nightcap on his head, and the demon-like nisus, it is hard to tell whether the classical form of the preformistic theory or the epigenetics theory was more naive.

Erikson's explanation of epigenesis is hardly more accurate than that of Jones. He states: "Freud showed that sexuality develops in stages, a *growth* which he firmly linked with all epigenetic development. . . . Embryology now understands epigenetic development, the step-by-step *growth* of fetal organs. . . . " (13, p.

61; italics mine). Erikson here also uses the idea of growth and thus implies an underlying preformism in terms of a preformed structure that grows. In the discussion from which this passage is drawn, Erikson tries to emphasize the novelty and importance of Freud's notion that sexual behavior in adolescence has antecedents. However, all that Freud actually accomplished was to move the moment of introduction of sexual interest in time from adolescence to infancy. It still grew, unfolding until it finally blossomed in adolescence; as such it is still a preformistic notion originating in innate givens.

Although Freud pushed the genetics of sexuality back in the life history of the individual, there is very little evidence to support the notion of an innate sexual drive that grows. As Beach puts it:

> To a much greater extent than is true of hunger or thirst, the sexual tendencies depend for their arousal upon external stimuli. The quasi-romantic [1] concept of the rutting stag actively seeking a mate is quite misleading. When he encounters a receptive female the male animal may or may not become sexually excited, but it is most unlikely that in the absence of erotic stimuli he exists in a constant state of undischarged sexual tensions. This would be equally true of the human male, were it not for the potent effects of symbolic stimuli which he tends to carry with him wherever he goes (14, p. 5).

Beach mixes his metaphors at the very end of the quote when he suggests that human males carry preformed imagery around with them. We could easily amend the statement to read epigenetically, in the sense used in this chapter, by adding merely that in the human, a wider range of stimuli not directly connected with a receptive female can activate the male. This is by no means exclusive to humans, as anyone who has been bothered by a dog mounting his leg can attest.

The spatial metaphor in the word *epigenetics* can be rescued. *Epi* can also be regarded as a spatial means of indicating a whole, the concept of a system rather than an individual thing. A psychophysiological illustration might clarify this notion. It has been observed that when we in the Western world watch a movie, we

---

1. The author's point that romantic love, a literary concept, has widely influenced science is well taken and deserves wider notice than can be given it in this chapter.

watch the whole picture, the *performance,* and not the individual items or things (15, p. 287). We do this by focusing slightly in front of the screen in a process that might be called "epi-focusing." When members of cultures unfamiliar with the movie-as-performance idea see a movie they are apt to focus, not slightly before the screen, but directly on it, where a specific object is shown. Consequently, the totality of the story and its message are missed. The *epi* in *epigenetics* parallels this psychophysiological "epi-focusing" in a similar effort to grasp the total performance. In addition to their failure to observe the totality of such an experience as a movie, members of non-Western cultures also differ from us in that there are situations where they do apply this form of observation but where we do not. For example, the Tlingit Indians were thought by Westerners to be crazy because they often sat for hours before the sea "in a trance," staring at the whole performance. When Westerners came upon them, they looked for something, some *thing,* on the sea. Failing to find anything on which to focus their vision and unable to focus on the totality, they declared the Tlingit Indians psychotic and named the syndrome after the tribe (16). Presumably, the Tlingits would feel the same way about the "trance" into which we go in the movies.

Epigenetics concerns itself with systems, with organizations, with events that are performances rather than objects or structures. Any discussion of the development or characteristics of a single entity cannot be epigenetic, since by definition a system or organization consists of at least two things standing in relationship to each other. The field of dance theory in contrast to theater may help to illustrate this point. With regard to drama we think in terms of roles, parts, entities that can exist offstage as well as on. But in dance, except in danced drama, we think almost entirely of the performance: a pas-de-deux, a leap, and so forth. A dancer's part off-stage no longer exists outside of the totality of the performance. It is in this sense that epigenetics is the study of systematic relationships that can be called performances.

RELEVANCE TO PSYCHOTHERAPY

Gill and Rapaport (17) note that there are implied throughout Freud's writing four basic assumptions related to his genetic formulations which might be profitably stated and discussed to further clarify the concept of epigenetics. As stated by Gill and Rapaport, they are:

1. All psychological phenomena have a psychological origin and development.

2. All psychological phenomena originate in innate givens, which mature according to an epigenetic ground plan.

3. The earlier forms of a psychological phenomenon, though superseded by later forms, remain potentially active.

4. At each point of psychological history the totality of potentially active earlier forms codetermines all subsequent psychological phenomena (17, p. 805).

It is particularly evident in the second assumption that the word *epigenetics* is being used inaccurately; it is associated with the concept of "innate givens," meaning either structure (homunculus) or invisible latent structure (anlage). But this is preformism as it became sophisticated soon after the homunculus idea was discarded. First, it is implied that the whole complexity of the organism is, in an *invisible form*, present in the ovum. Secondly, this visible or invisible structure grows or matures according to a "ground plan" which we presumably know already. This notion is based on a natural history time concept. Third, the "epigenetic" seems to mean in this context that the rate of development is determined by a pacemaker, by another structure. We may note that transferring the problem of genetics, narrowly defined as an issue of rate, to another structure called a pacemaker, leaves unanswered the question that applied to the original structure: namely, how did *it* develop? This, in turn, might be explained by another pacemaker for the pacemaker—an explanation that in logic is called an infinite regress.

To understand the significance of these assumptions, especially the last two (3 and 4), we must recognize the basic problem with which Freud had to cope. He was regularly confronted with the argument or criticism that his theories applied only to special cases such as degenerates, and did not have reference to people in general. Freud's genetic theories were designed to counteract this criticism, to construct a psychology of the species and not of a few peculiar individuals. But many of his important ideas, such as that of the unconscious, were virtually impossible to demonstrate convincingly. For example, he wanted to make it clear that the content of the unconscious is species-wide, but by definition this material never enters our awareness and we can never directly know what it is. To use evidence about the unconscious derived from what comes to the surface in nightmares or psychosis does not mean that the findings really apply to the majority of people who are normal. This would be as fallacious as claiming that malarial parasites are species-wide on the basis of a study only of malaria patients.

Freud sought to bolster his claims about the universality of the unconscious with the assumptions stated above. First he asserted the existence of a psychological universe: all psychological phenomena are given to all people in the same innate form. Second, these innate givens develop according to a fixed "ground plan" that can vary only in terms of pace. Third, it is assumed that the earlier forms remain either potentially or actively influential. This, in effect, inverts the earlier preformistic idea by saying that the tree is a grown-up acorn: for the acorn to be able to influence the mature oak, it must in some sense still be that acorn. In short then, taken together, these assumptions establish a species-wide psychology, which was Freud's major intention.

In spite of a certain lack of clarity, there is a *double* preformism in Freud's genetics with which we have to deal. First, there is a preformed structure, and second, a preformed series of stages through which this structure grows. To fully differentiate epigenetics from preformism we must therefore speak of a double epigenetics in which structure is replaced by network or system, and in which natural history's preformed stages are replaced by a cyclical model of time. Preformism postulates an end point in its time model, a final form, structure, or stage. As social psychiatrists come to devote increasing attention to the life span after adolescence, emphasis has shifted to a time model which is cyclical: the family life cycle. While we may arbitrarily interrupt the cyclical loop for discussion purposes, there is no final stage or form that evolves.

Preformism and epigenetics represent, respectively, psychoanalytic and social psychiatric theory. In this framework it is seen that they vary in terms of their generalizations. Preformism in Freudian genetics was adopted to promote the idea of a universal or species-wide psychology. Epigenetics signifies for social psychiatry a psychology of circumstances, a pluralism in terms of which behavior is assumed to vary according to a field or network of events. In theory the distinction may seem somewhat esoteric, but there are direct practical consequences stemming from each assumption. For example, in selection procedures, the Freudian would apply a single standard of overall psychological adjustment in choosing naval recruits for such diverse tasks as submarine duty or maintenance of isolated posts in the South Pole. Social psychiatrists, however, would use specific criteria for each situation, preferably defined by people who had been there. It has in fact been found in many assessment situations that the most successful candidates for such unusual assignments are not necessarily the most well-adjusted (in the Freudian's sense), but possess quirks and peculiarities which make them comfortable in unusual environments.

Another consequence of this theoretical distinction concerns the sources selected for study in cases of abnormal or atypical behavior. The psychoanalyst, and indeed most psychiatrists trained in traditional settings, typically adopted a historian's viewpoint in their search for what went wrong, and investigate events of the past to see in what way they may have brought about the present situation. In his novel *Cards of Identity*, Nigel Dennis illustrates in satirical terms how this historical orientation of psychoanalysis combines with a species-wide psychology:

> When I first joined this club our great theory was in a fluid condition. So, in consequence, was my identity. We had to build both our case-histories and autobiographies upon patients who showed promise of corroboration. But as the theory grew stronger, so did the patient become more and more superfluous. . . . We rebelled against servitude to men and women whose condition had been diagnosed to perfection years before they ever entered our consulting room. . . . We all felt like dentists who had created plates or bridges of pure gold to the most cunning design and were obliged to sit and wait for the appropriate jaws to come in. We were as judges who had already pronounced sentence; only the criminal remained at a distance . . . (18, pp. 139–140).

In sharp contrast, the social psychiatrist studies the present rather than the past. Since he rejects the metaphors of inner space, affect, and the unconscious, in favor of behavior, he is not concerned with the Oedipus *complex* but with what to do for Oedipus himself, the man. If we consider Job as another representation of tragedy, we can see the irrelevance of historical explanation to his current predicament. In the course of his misfor tunes, three friends come to him and try to help by encouraging a historical reconstruction of events to locate the sinful or "abnormal" behavior which they presume brought about his trials. Job ultimately rejects their efforts and turns his attention again to the present problem. In this myth, the social psychiatrist is more concerned with the initial argument between God and the devil about the extent to which men can remain autonomous from their social and physical circumstances. In other terms, the issue is one of the nature of courage, the strictly moral question of how one can stay on the course one has set for oneself under stress, that is, maintain cyclical behavior. For social psychiatrists, the task involves not going back into the past for sequential or historical explanation, but considering the current array of influences. It would be tempting to say that the issue is to go not back to the past but forward to the future; however, this alternative is really a modification of the same linear point of view of the historian. Rather, the problems of Oedipus and Job translated into modern social psychiatry become for the psychiatrist the management and repair of disaster.

Application of the historical perspective to events represents a strong if invisible form of influence on them. In a sense there is no such thing as a neutral historian. Since it would be utterly impossible to recount every single past incident, some selection process is inevitable, and in this way if in no other the historian shapes his material. More often his influence is less subtle, and his restatements of the past are specifically intended to have some kind of impact on the present. The same applies to predictions of events to come. To be told one's future is as much a manipulation of the present as to be told one's past. In education as in psychotherapy, the phenomenon of the self-fulfilling prophecy has been amply documented.

Historical accounts can provide propaganda material or ideological fuel to support some contemporary political or cultural program. The relativism inherent in histories becomes clear when we compare two accounts of the same period, originating at different times. For example, the American frontier of the nineteenth century was long presented as the epitome of democracy, where hardworking pioneers were rewarded with free land and other governmental help. Today, in a milieu of militant civil rights campaigns, this past is being reexamined and is now being seen as an era of perpetuation of racial inequality, since the vast majority of the pioneers who received these benefits were white.

Contemporary interests also direct the attention of historians to periods, places, and qualities in the past that had hitherto been ignored. As Mead noted, "every great social movement has flashed back its light to discover a new past" (19, p. 62). Continuing with the example of the effect of current interest in civil rights on history, it is observable that there exists today a new and active interest in African Negro history. This has created new fields of study and a new cast of characters, such as the African chief who once ruled a territory larger than that of the United States.

These observations apply to the description of an individual's history as well as to the pasts of groups or nations. In the course of cataloguing, the historian inevitably influences the present by his selection of past events. Application of the historical framework virtually compels one to search for explanations of current behavior in the past, instead of examining the ongoing situation for relevant factors. Thus when a therapist says, "There must be some reason in your past to account for your fight with your wife last night," he is largely negating the possibility of any legitimate present reason, such as the wife's behavior, and suggesting that the patient does not come by his fight honestly. As another example, Goffman (20) has shown that the case-history construction of events in clinical practice often casts doubt on the patient's adequacy as a human being from childhood on, even if he is being psychiatrically examined for the first time at the age of fifty. This reinterpretation of the past can serve as a device for making more palatable for their next of kin the hospitalization of people who are *currently* irritating, by implying that all their lives they had been getting sick until their illness became so bad that they now require hospitalization for their own sake. Perhaps these examples can show that when psychiatrists "take" a history they are exerting great influence on the present set of circumstances. In this sense a history is not an initial step in diagnosis but one of the many power operations that can be used by patient and therapist to influence present events.

The social psychiatrist is concerned with a performance. A performance by definition consists of many simultaneous events and cannot have a linear history. At most a performance may have had previous cycles, and perhaps an accumulated smoothness or polish from repeated rehearsals. When something goes wrong, the social psychiatrist searches for concurrent events that may be relevant. He is like a detective, not a historian. He searches, not in the past for a traumatic event or disturbance, but in the ongoing situation. The detective analogy is quite helpful in explaining the approach of the social psychiatrist. If the initial or presenting complaint is seen as the first clue, the detective then searches for the "crime" by collecting as many observations as possible. For example, a child brought for treatment can be seen as the instigation for an investigation into the workings of the family and its relations with society. It becomes quickly apparent that the initial complaint or problem was a simplified version of a complex pattern of simultaneously occurring events: in other words, a performance, which is not now working smoothly. It is not easily typed, and there is no single solution that becomes obvious once the diagnosis is made. Instead, some construction of events is formulated by the social psychiatrist; it is discussed, fought over and modified by the participants, and finally an agreement is reached on some course of action. Hopefully, the regularity or pattern of the performance is reestablished.

The social psychiatrist thus thinks about a complexity of contexts impinging on each other: family, job, social network. He does not consider the presence of preexisting disease in one family member any more than the law entertains the notion of preexisting criminality in a defendant in court. Otherwise the law would not insist that each time a man appears in court he is to be treated as if newly accused. There are no entities such as mental patients or criminals: just judgments by others which are perpetually fallible.

You cannot pick a criminal and you cannot pick a patient and you cannot pick a dandelion, because they are not structural entities with careers independent of their contexts. A dandelion isn't a thing; it's a performance. And you know, every living thing is a performance, even you. The dandelion is that segment of the performance, the process, which lasts, which slows down to such a snail's pace that we see it as a thing. . . .

CHAPTER SIX

Energy: Economics

Son: How do geese know to fly south?
Father: They are led by instinct.
Son: Is he the one who flies in front?

The concept of an instinctual psychic energy organizes in a single doctrine the notions that have been discussed in previous chapters: inner space, the unconscious, preformism, and imponderables.

Inner space is a prerequisite for the concept of psychic energy because the energy is seen as residing within the organism. Freud started out, notably in the 1895 *Project for a Scientific Psychology* (1), to develop a mechanical explanation of the individual mind. Although this effort was not successful, he did not turn to a purely psychological model, as is sometimes thought, but continued to follow the doctrine of the famous physiologist du Bois-Reymond (1842): "No other forces than the common physical-chemical ones are active within the organism. In those cases which cannot at the time be explained by these forces one has either to find a specific way or form of their action by means of the physical-mathematical method, *or to assume new forces* equal in dignity to the chemical-physical forces inherent in matter, reducible to the force of attraction and repulsion" (2. Italics mine). Because Freud's notion of psychic energy was intended to be ultimately reunited with anatomy and physiology, it was patterned on what was known at the time about the brain. He did not want to construct a purely academic psychology, however, any more than he wished to err in the other direction long popular in the history of science, which was known as vitalism and which implied mystical and supernatural forces. To avoid either of these extremes, Freud created what is sometimes called a brain mythology, in which the ultimate goal was to conceive of the mind as a machine and energy as the fuel. By deciding to place the residence of the events he studied within the mind, however, Freud's theorizing about energy concepts became basically vitalistic even though his goal was a physiological model. If he had not invoked the concept of inner space, the domain to be studied would concern the transactions of two or more physiologies with other elements in the environment. Thus, rather than follow du Bois-Reymond's dictum and apply physiological ideas to a mythical mental organ, it becomes more relevant to modify his advice by turning to another branch of science, ecology, which will be discussed below.

In conjunction with the concept of unconscious purpose in mental life, psychic energy inserts teleological formulations into psychology. It is not the *fact* of goal-direction that is questionable, but an explanation that presumes an *unanalyzable* category of purpose, a principle or force that seeks or supplies the fuel that drives the organism toward the goal. Cybernetics, for instance, does not require teleological reasoning, and it provides a satisfactory description of purposive behavior based on concepts utilizing information theory. Psychic energy, in contrast, is teleological in the sense that it is directional, has an aim which can be modified only with difficulty, and is often described in crudely anthropomorphic terms: it "struggles," "presses for discharge," is "ever on the alert for opportunities," and so forth (3).

The unconscious serves as a transition to a preformistic notion of "executive causality." The idea that there is a mechanical substrate driven by an *executive pacemaker* which also serves as a source of power is completely compatible with modern vitalistic theory. Driesch (1867–1941), known as the last major spokesman for vitalism within science, called himself "a consistent mechanist" precisely because he did not object to a mechanical and extreme preformistic view but merely proposed a vital force called entelechy which he conceptualized as the engineer who set the machine in motion. The concept of imponderables further complicates the picture, although within psychology it is an anachronistic survival of premechanical notions. However, to the extent that psychology conceives of the mind as a mechanism with a fuel tank, it is vulnerable to the habits of thought and language which insert imponderables into such containers, and makes difficult the elimination of such simplistic or misleading notions.

Seventy years after Freud started to work on the problem of a brain model it has become apparent that neither the mechanistic nor vitalistic points of view are helpful; mechanical notions fail because they attempt to view the subject matter of psychiatry as exclusively physiological or physiochemical, and the vitalistic approach fails because of its concern with speculative, philosophical, and supernatural causes. Psychic energy is thus an untenable theoretical entity which rests on a flawed set of concepts discussed in earlier chapters and, moreover, leads to basically spiritualistic answers. Ironically, Freud's energy concepts have long attracted attention because they appear to be more "scientific" and potentially measurable than many other psychoanalytic concepts. Ostow (4) has referred to psychic energy as the only quantitative concept that Freud introduced, and several unsuccessful efforts have been made to measure it (3). This unjustified "scientific" appearance of psychic energy is partly due to the tendency of individual psychology to postulate an inner world, a mythic domain in which processes are assumed to transpire which correspond to those in the real world of the laboratory scientist. When electricity, for instance, was thought to coat pith balls with a charge in the outside world, a mental electricity (psychic energy) was postulated to coat (cathect) memory traces in the world within. Even if the precision of the physicist was not immediately applicable to psychoanalysis in practice, it appeared to be in principle. This approach has become discredited and has resulted in the odd juxtaposition of men calling themselves scientists yet accommodating overtly spiritualistic doctrines. Freud, for instance, believed in telepathy. In order to understand how this paradox has come about, we must examine the demands made on psychology within the Western cultural tradition.

The scientific explanation of a bone fracture in Galilean terms (consideration of the vectorial forces on the bones, resistance of the bones, and so forth) does not explain *why* the fracture happened to a particular victim at a given time. It is critically important to recognize that the scientific method can never answer such "why" questions without ceasing to be scientific. Even with the cybernetic alternative to teleology, all that science can offer is an infinite series of causes. Questions concerning purpose, motivation, and responsibility demand consideration of an *executive* causality that is not within the province of our scientific tradition. It is generally agreed that "the study of purpose in Nature is inconsistent with the scientific aim, which is the adequate description of phenomena" (5, p. 385). Other cultures may conceive of the scientific method somewhat differently; thus an association of African witch doctors, comparing the craft of its members with that of Western medicine, commented that the latter can only tell *what* causes a disease while a witch doctor can reveal the equally important considerations of *who* and *why*. From this standpoint it can be argued that true prevention, as opposed to "merely cure," must deal with why a disease happened as well as with its scientific causes. While this assertion can be questioned, it does highlight the fact that many psychological explanations rest on concepts that block inquiry into the origins of a problem by postulating categories said to be unanalyzable by definition, and therefore block efforts at prevention. This point will be extended in a later discussion.

Newton's scientific breakthrough, his really astonishing departure, was to stop asking "why" questions and to focus instead on the description of events and phenomena (this is not to say that he answered the "why" questions before dismissing them). This radical change in method and outlook is usually presented by reference to Newton's famous dictum, *hypothesis non fingo* (literally: I invent no hypothesis). The meaning of the term *hypothesis* has changed since Newton's day, which has led to common errors in the translation of this dictum. Newton meant "thing placed under" when he referred to *hypothesis*. The phrase was intended to indicate that he conceived of a world entirely in terms of science, totally independent of the medieval and Christian views that predominated until then. He "had conceived a working universe wholly independent of the spiritual order" (5, p. 294); he put nothing "under" his mechanical system, particularly not the energy concepts associated with vitalism and spiritualism. The Newtonian viewpoint thus replaced the old cosmology with a world view in which the teleological questions raised today were no longer asked.

Newton introduced the age of scientific determinism around 1700; his work marks the beginnings of modern scientific theory and method. It seems at first gratuitous to inquire whether the principles he espoused are universally accepted by today's scientists, and yet some reflection indicates the relevance of this question for psychiatry. Has psychiatry indeed relinquished all interest in "why" questions, or are issues of responsibility, purpose, and motivation inextricably bound to many of its contemporary doctrines? To return to the example of the bone fracture mentioned earlier, does the psychoanalytic notion of "accident proneness," formulated as an unconscious source of energy directed toward hurting oneself, express a scientific formulation, or does it represent a modern format of the old basically spiritualistic question? The entire concept of mind (whether conscious or unconscious) as *responsible* via psychic energy for acts or events brings the psychoanalytic point of view uncomfortably close to the medieval concept of soul. Dewey stated this categorically: "The 'mind' as 'actor' . . . is the old self-acting 'soul.' . . . It has always been a bit of a mystery as to just how the commonplace 'soul' of the Middle Ages . . . came to blossom out into the overstrained, tense and morbid 'psyche' of the last two centuries" (6, p. 131). Indeed, the notion that an act is committed on purpose by an unconscious agency is so similar in form (if not always in content) to a spiritualistic personification that it is merely reversed in metaphoric location—one deep and the other transcendental—but both depart from the center of the target, which for social phychiatry is the transactions in natural groups.

Through most of its history, psychology has sought the stature and proprieties of being considered scientific, but this has proved an elusive goal. Many concepts that seem scientific merely mask a spiritualism with science's metaphors and mystique. Holt (3) states that the concepts of energy and force were so important to the nineteenth-century mechanistic world view that their use in Freud's time was virtually a hallmark of science. Psychic energy became a vitalistic or even spiritualistic wolf in the sheep's clothing of physiological science. Social psychiatry seeks to avoid the pitfalls of either, and as such must reject both the mechanistic and vitalistic points of view; the subject matter of social psychiatry is neither the occult nor the physiological, but is far more compatible with the disciplines of ecology or embryology which we will consider next.

THE EMBRYOLOGY OF BEHAVIOR

We no longer accept the notion of spontaneous generation, that a maggot is created by the sun's rays in a piece of rotten meat. We now know that the maggot is a fly larva and that a fly has laid a microscopic egg on the meat. In the study of behavior, however, the following dichotomies are similar in form and effect to the concept of spontaneous generation in the sense that they block inquiry into the origins of the behavior under consideration:

> instinct—habit
> innate—acquired
> unlearned—learned
> nature—nurture
> genetic—environmental

Psychic energy serves as a companion to such patterns of thought. Once a category or specific bit of behavior is seen as unprecedented, one cannot inquire into its origins—its embryology, so to speak—and it is considered preformed. It is subsequently seen as a mechanism which is driven by an energy. The African witch doctors can then complain, as we have noted, that prevention is impossible in the Western scheme of things, since this requires knowledge of antecedents.

Erroneous language habits encourage us to think in terms of the instinctual-noninstinctual dichotomy. This error has been exposed by Ginsberg (7) in his examination of the logic of such dichotomies. He refers to eight major logical fallacies, including a failure to define what is meant by "innate." In most cases the term is defined on the basis of ignorance: that which is not understood (at least at present) is, by process of elimination, assumed to be innate. If we do not understand what makes up a complex behavioral sequence such as leg-raising in a male dog, we can cover our ignorance, and incidentally block further inquiry into the behavior's origins, by assigning it to a mechanical "urinary instinct" which is powered by a so-called reaction-specific energy. The developmental perspective is short-circuited conceptually at this point. When a dog is found who does not raise his leg, we are left to conclude that the urinary instinct or the energy is deficient, not that a complex series of antecedents failed to take place which, if we know more about, we might be able to induce correctively later on.

Schneirla has said that " 'innateness' is nothing more than a poor hypothesis" (8, p. 287). Somewhat analogously, Holt has suggested that psychic energy has played no part in generating empirical studies, "however long it may linger in the . . . atmosphere of the clinic" (3) as a way of talking about phenomena. Such explanations have the apparent advantage of appearing physiological because of the mechanical language involved, yet they are all basically container-ingredient models, which, as we have seen in earlier chapters, bias our language system. Instead of being a bottle, the container is now a machine and the ingredient a fuel-like energy. The basic model, however, is not significantly different from the mind-imponderable model used for centuries. In this sense acquired or learned behavior represents subjects about which we have some knowledge, and instinctive, unlearned or innate behavior refers to that about which we are currently ignorant.[1]

In summary, the concept of psychic energy is a poor hypothesis which survives because it fits well into our container-ingredient language, protects us from acknowledging ignorance, and incorrectly misleads the scientist into believing that his thinking is potentially physiological or mechanistic when in fact he is courting the less attractive alternative of spiritualism or vitalism. It is unfortunate that the possibility of an ecological or embryological

1. In other usage, such terms as *innate* refer to typical behavior of a species. However, when *instinctive behavior* is used that way care must be taken to emphasize that it is merely descriptive of "a range of behavior functions that develop under conditions more or less typical of the species" (8, p. 287).

approach is not more often seen as a solution to this dilemma. In psychiatry a reevaluation of all aspects of metapsychology is required, in view of the interrelationships between the concepts of psychic energy, imponderables, the unconscious, preformism, and the topic of the next chapter—structure.

Even if such reevalutation is undertaken, a new perspective is adopted in terms of which we no longer consider problems as residing within the individual, and we are able to attend to the embryology of behavior and the ecology of the environment, we find that the same confusing mixture of spiritualism and physiological concepts have preceded us there for the very reasons that we have been discussing.

PHYSIOLOGY VERSUS ECOLOGY

The physiological or economic point of view pervades current social ideologies. "Justice triumphs," "truth will out," "love conquers all" are all simple, popular, and appealing expressions derived from a model of society in which the unanalyzable forces represented by or behind love, justice, and truth "naturally" lead to the conditions observed. While these slogans are trite, at the other end of the spectrum one finds the same basically physiological approach applied to even the most complex and sophisticated descriptions of pathology. Even in current terms, when game theory is used to describe normal or deviant behavior, a force is frequently postulated which is said to find for itself a clever means of satisfaction although the participants might protest that they are suffering terribly. Even if they state that their intentions are the converse of their current transactions, some mysterious *physiology* or *energy* is seen as being *in equilibrium*. Although the game framework is more descriptive than a statement of motives, something is missing in this type of interpretation.

It is a step in the right direction to suggest actual behavior in a game theory framework rather than bare motives powered by the workings of a teleological energy. The metaphor "roulette" is more descriptive of certain behavior than "an energy striving to achieve forbidden goals" applied to the same transaction. However, except in the case of the actual game of roulette the descrip-

tion of behavior leaves something to be desired. The real roulette
player, whatever his motive, has the freedom to enter and leave
the game. One follows the rules of a game in a different sense
than one follows the laws of physiology. One can say metaphorically that the actual game of roulette has an artificial economy or
physiology. However, once we venture from the actual player in
the actual game to a pathological gambler or a professional gambler, one who illegally earns his living in the activity, the rules of
the game that describe the artificial economy or physiology do
not apply. Additional theoretical material must be added to adequately explain the situation, let alone the transaction in which
roulette is used in a purely metaphoric sense. Even if a new game
is invented which includes the pathological gambler's game, another game must be invented to explain entry and involvement
in *that* game. The games needed to adequately describe the situation become infinite in number and increasingly complex. To describe the alternative to such physiological notions, whether simple or complex, criticism of the underlying physiological, economic, or equilibrium model is necessary.

THRASYMACHUS' ARGUMENT

There is a remarkable argument in the first book of Plato's *Republic* which expresses for the first time in recorded history a severe criticism of the physiological model.

Socrates is journeying home from Piraeus, the port of Athens,
from a religious ceremony and festival when he is overtaken by a
group of acquaintances who insist, jokingly, we are told, that they
will not let him go home. He must join them to supply some en-
tertaining conversation. The first result is a polite discussion with
the elder, Cephalus, about wisdom and old age. Cephalus states
rather immodestly that he is content in his old age because he has
been just, and implies that because he has been just, the world
has been just to him. The basic idea is a physiological one. Justice is a force or energy which can be stored and drawn upon, but
it cannot be further analyzed or brought under natural science
considerations. It is, in fact, supernatural. Cephalus is pompous
and fatuous, but in seeking to deny other causes for his comforta-

ble old age, he does reveal that he was born rich and powerful.

The excitement of the writing is contained not within the content of the argument but rather within the meager plot, although it is clear to all readers that this is intended as a fabric with which to hold the philosophical dialogue together. However, in the plot Socrates' presence there seems not so much an outcome of justice, whatever that is, but rather of thinly disguised brute force. We are *not* told that Socrates owed a debt to Cephalus for some just action—rather Polemachus, the son of Cephalus, says (jokingly, of course) when he catches up with Socrates, that his cronies are many and Socrates one—and that therefore Socrates had better join them. He is all but dragged into the house, although admittedly he begins to enjoy his stay. We might at this point wonder what Xanthippe, Socrates' wife, who is the prototypical shrewish woman, will have to say about his lateness, and whether he is not under some obligation to get home. In point of fact the setting that Plato sketches for the discussion to follow is therefore not in keeping with Cephalus' point of view.

Socrates responds with the question, "What, after all, is justice?" For a moment it looks as though Socrates is going to expose the old hypocrite, but the latter ducks out to participate in a religious ceremony and his son continues the discussion for a while, with Socrates arriving at no very profound conclusions.

One of the company can contain himself no longer, forgets his manners, and blurts out, "Socrates, what kind of nonsense are you blabbing about all the time?"

"Justice," says Thrasymachus, "is the utility of the stronger." Thrasymachus does not lose the ensuing argument. He seems to sense that Socrates is more powerful, that any continuation of the argument will irritate his powerful hosts, and, true to his own theory, demurs. The whole argument resembles a dominance fight among animals. When it becomes clear that Socrates will be supported by the pack, Thrasymachus becomes submissive. This is not the interpretation that Plato intends, of course. He would prefer that Thrasymachus be seen as rude, intemperate, prideful —all those qualities which for the Greeks were the opposite of logical. But if Plato cannot support him in his dialogue, he does so within the plot. The behavior of the people within the story appears to be the outcome of their response to power. If this is a useful principle applicable to social transactions in general, then perhaps it is possible to analyze justice further than Socrates would acknowledge. Thrasymachus' suggestion is that those in power establish rules and sanctions that essentially benefit and are useful to them. These rules are called by them just. Justice is therefore "the utility of the stronger."

Part of the problem with supporting or even fully understanding Thrasymachus in his presentation is the overwhelming number of problems set him all at once. The issue is focused not by disputing the nature of justice but by a broader dispute about the nature of the social world—whether it is to be seen as physiological or ecological. Do beauty, truth, justice, and so forth reveal themselves as a result of an energy that they contain which overcomes the resistances to them, or are these terms merely the labels applied to the winning side of a struggle? The issue has many practical consequences. For instance, if justice is self-evident then we should endorse the idea that juries should be unanimous because truth is easily seen by all. On the other hand, if it is always a matter of a struggle, perhaps the old Judaic notion that juries should have a hard time deciding their verdict is correct. In the latter case unanimity of a jury is a sought-after condition because it is difficult to achieve; here the danger lies in too easy a decision because this would reveal merely a defect in the prosecution or the defense, not justice. If a decision is handed down quickly, the sides must have been poorly matched. If, on the other hand, we follow Socrates (Plato), such a decision is the result of obvious truth and justice.

We have, on the one hand, a "Machiavellian approach" which exposes conflict and the exercise of power against resistance as a principle for the understanding of social and environmental processes, and, on the other hand, a "Rousseauan approach" which implies a social organization, a general will or consensus of values. The former point of view is ecological and the latter physiological. For the physiologist those in power act as agents of the corporate social body or organism. No one is seen as devoid of power. All citizens participate in making the system work. Fairness and justice, like respiration and digestion, are concepts that help to explain the functioning of the organism.

There are emotional connotations to such a dichotomy. At first the ecological or Machiavellian emphasis appears close to a description of a totalitarian dictatorship. On the other hand, such supposed benevolence as implied by the physiological approach is obviously inhospitable to dynamic change, and, if it is wrong, can be seen as the ideology of stagnation and suppression held by those who wish to think of themselves as benevolent.

Strategies of intervention in consulting or treating natural groups differ, depending upon whether the entry is made from an ecological or physiological point of view. When a social psychiatrist approaches a natural system such as a school or a police unit, he is concerned with his political support and attempts to make an entry and work from a position of power, from the top. On the other hand, a physiological theorist is less inclined to actively solicit support from those in power and thinks more in terms of a consensus from the social body. The most common error in working with natural groups within the community is to obtain access to the lowest-ranking members (schoolteachers or patrolmen) and consult with them. The alternative is to work with the entire natural group, including all those in power (for instance, principals, teachers, and handymen), with the focus upon the transactions between them.

HUMAN ECOLOGY

The ecological point of view is one in which the key concepts of the physiological approach can be further analyzed in terms of the dynamics of power and resistance. It rejects in particular those notions of unanalyzable energy or power that are usually assigned to a mythical social organism rather than to clusters of people. It is tempting to say that the ecological approach is basically "political," except that even here one frequently hears of mythical monsters such as the military-industrial complex, which is spoken of as if it were a social organism in which every person in the military and every businessman participated, rather than simply a coalition of a few influential people. On the level of the family, the physiological approach postulates an organism, while the ecological approach postulates that a family is an environment with an ecology no more obscurely bounded by a theoretical skin than a pasture, a lake, or a "biome" like the Arctic.

The choice between a physiological point of view and an ecological one is crucial to all subsequent thought. Classification can be taken as an example. Animals are classified by their relationship to evolution. Environments can be classified in relationship to the process of *succession,* an ecological concept with many similarities to evolution. Networks of living and non-living objects (or simply environments) slowly change towards a "climax state" in which a stable condition prevails and is maintained by climax forces unless some catastrophe occurs. Lakes turn into ponds and ponds into bogs and bogs into swamps. Swamps dry up and become meadows, then thickets, and thousands of years later climax forests. The character of the entire series of steps is determined by general conditions of height, rainfall, climate, and so forth. In the Arctic and in the tropics the successive steps undergone by a lake vary at least in terms of rates and specific species. The more general conditions map out biomes, areas that tend to have the same climax conditions. Any particular environment can have a set of names, just as any animal can, and there is no theoretical limit to how small a unit can be classified. A log on the forest floor is a micro-environment which also undergoes this process of succession.

In an article written in 1916, Robert E. Park attempted to utilize ecology in relation to human behavior in the urban environment (9). Park suggested that cities, like other large areas, had within them "natural areas" in which people with similar social, ethnic, and economic backgrounds were segregated. He divided the city of Chicago into what were to become seventy-five natural areas for purposes of study. This approach has sparked a series of ecological studies of humans as well as the branch of study known as urban sociology.

Human behavior seems to vary within different environments. Personalities can be defined as parts of such environments and should therefore submit to ecological classification. For instance, certain tropical climates support a variety of poverty that cannot be supported in the Arctic or the arid desert. Schizophrenia is found in high proportion in the disorganized communities near the centers of cities. The inner city area may produce an unusual number of schizophrenics, or they might drift into such areas. The different hypotheses are asking essentially the same ecological question: "Why do certain conditions bring about a high concentration of a certain phenomenon?" The question is ecological in nature, and the answer may eventually be provided by a "new biology."

Beginning steps have been made in expanding this general approach on such matters as climate and mental health, architecture and mental health, and the work of conservationists who actively argue that their work is not for the preservation of odd species but for the preservation of environments which include *Homo sapiens.*

Most of the basic research on the process of succession in the networks that include humans has yet to be done. The result would be a classification scheme which would describe the hysteric personality, for instance, in terms of the nature of the micro-environment around such a person rather than in terms of what happens to the distribution of energy. While ecology and field biology are comparatively young sciences in relation to experimental biology, some of the groundwork has been done, including agreement on sampling techniques, units of measurement, and general classes and subdomains within a nomenclature of classes. This provides some basis for agreement regarding the expected course of events and therefore some notion of relative health and deviance from norms. As far as human networks or environments are concerned even these preliminary steps have not been accomplished, and it would be incorrect to imply that the hysteric personality or any other has been already mapped in relationship to an environment. Limited clinical observations of the hysteric suggest a rather barren environment. Other observations on conversion reaction suggest the presence of certain important relationships to medical institutions (10). Observations of delinquents indicate other sets of complex interrelationships (11). As more of these descriptions are accumulated and related to ecological theory a classification scheme will evolve.

Ecology has little use for the energy concepts of physiological social theory. The so-called great chain of life supplies the only necessary energy concepts in ecological theory. The sun's energy is utilized by plants which are eaten by vegetarians who, in turn, are eaten by carnivores who eventually die and supply energy to plants. It has never seemed necessary to explain simple or complex behavior in the environment by something further than this energy. When a carnivore eats a vegetarian, that activity (eating) is related to the chain of energy already discussed, not to some new form of power within the carnivore.

RELEVANCE TO PSYCHOTHERAPY

For the most part, psychotherapists utilize a home gardening analogy rather than an ecological point of view in thinking about their work. They see themselves as being charged with the task of growing something like a rare plant under greenhouse conditions. In a rather polyannish way they view their job as the watering and care, the nurturing of an organism until it flowers. No farmer would subscribe to such an approach with his crops beset by insects, natural disasters, fickle weather, and, finally, insecure market conditions—all of which he fights vigorously. However, it is not uncommon to read that the therapist merely "allows" a growth tendency, "a drive toward self-actualization, or a forward-moving directional tendency" (12, p. 35) to express itself. Such assertions and the gardening metaphor rest on the vitalistic notion of psychic energy already discussed. The therapist and the naive gardener both postulate that the object in their charge has within it a preformed mechanism and an executive pacemaker which is the real object of their care. It is this unseen object that must be nurtured until it flourishes. Since such growth in the case of humans is seen as powered by psychic energy, the therapist sees his job as freeing more of it for growth purposes. Such a therapist tends to think of himself in the most benevolent terms. His area of operation is not with humans in the environment but rather in inner space, where there is already a goal or direction he merely assists somewhat. Any ecological assertion that implies another source of direction is declared manipulative and unethical.

The highest standards of ethics should be applied to the psychotherapeutic profession. About that there can be no quarrel. However, if the vitalistic notions of psychic energy and the cluster of concepts surrounding it (the unconscious, preformism, imponderables, inner space) are not applicable, a new perspective on ethics must be developed. The problem rests with the manipulative-nurturing dichotomy. If there is no inner space containing a direction, psychotherapeutic goals are set by people and "nurturing" is not a feasible posture. One must set ethical standards in relation to the use of power to attain goals and not deny that power is being used.

There are times when a therapist is frankly manipulative. In a recent case a female therapist was faced with a network of people which included a young adult whose favorite maneuver was to act crazy and, for instance, take off all his clothes. The therapist started off the first session by stating that she had heard that the young man performed when groups got together and therefore she would be happy to give him ten minutes right at the outset for him to do so. He started to act crazy; this time he crawled around on the floor and ate paper cups. However, it must be noticed that he did so at the therapist's request. When the ten minutes were up, the therapist said that it was time to stop and start the session, which he did. In the next session the therapist suggested that the performance should last five minutes, as there was a lot to take up from the last session. In this fashion the crazy symptoms were soon under the control of the therapist and could not serve a disruptive function. The rug was pulled out from under the young man rather adroitly. The therapist made no effort to explain, interpret, or nurture. She openly did battle with the most obvious troublemaker right at the outset. It is hard to view the process as anything but a power struggle and the therapist's task as other than a police function, to restore some semblance of law and order, give and take, to the group. Were the disruptive behavior actively assaultive, the situation would be more obvious. It would then follow that to have a session, peace would have to be restored. However, if it is possible to acknowledge that there is *psychic* brute force as well as physical brute force, an ethical justification for the therapist's behavior is possible.

The decision to act in this fashion was the therapist's. One could deviously hide such goal choice by implying that there was a secret direction similar to the one the therapist chose within the inner space of the group or the individual, that such behavior was a cry for help from a hidden homunculus. There are some therapists who, while acknowledging that such a maneuver is theoretically false, insist it is necessary politically in order to be more effective. These therapists are obscurely manipulative. They frequently view the family or the individual as a dangerous wild animal or pack who must be out-tricked and out-maneuvered at every stage of therapy. They feel the therapist's job is to double-bind the double-binders in order to free the patient from torture at his family's hands. Lately such therapists have been surprised to find that the patient is not always delighted by such release. He does not escape from the supposed trap the moment he is freed; in fact, he returns for more. It has become, therefore, harder to find a victim to support in such a situation. Thus the justification for "undercover" work is harder to support. A distinction therefore must be made between the therapist who is powerful and openly acknowledges it and the therapist who does the same things but disguises his power from his patients (and sometimes himself). The former is doing his job; the latter is also making an assault on the cognitive powers of his clients but creating confusing smokescreens that hide his motives and his techniques. One of the most obvious deleterious effects is that it is hard to learn from such a therapist since there is a disparity between what he does and what he says he does. After all, what lasting good is achieved if a therapist can deal sanely with a child but his parents cannot learn to do the same? Even in the situation in which a husband comes to a therapist alone for individual therapy, the therapist must form some evaluation of the marriage. When and if the marriage breaks up, he has had a hand in it, either to speed its demise or to retard it. When the couple splits up and the therapist has an anxiety attack, the advocate role of the therapist and the ethics involved become more obvious to him.

It is also possible to avoid being placed in manipulative positions by patients. "My daughter is behaving weirdly. Do something, doctor," is a frank appeal to a therapist to exert power which may or may not be ethical. On the other hand, "My daughter is behaving weirdly, what should her father and I do?" is an entirely different question. In individual therapy, "I have a psychiatric symptom, do something," is similar to the first request. In such a situation the Machiavellian position, the position of consultant to an individual or a natural group, appears to be more ethical and less manipulative than that in which one is hired by one member of a family to support him or by an individual to act as an alter ego.

The therapist enters, not to doctor an organism, to maintain a homeostatic system, or to nurture individual development, but rather to serve as a consultant or an advocate. The lawyer is frequently in the same position. In court, the slogan over the door may read, "The just man need not fear"; a defense attorney, however, is seeking not to reveal impartial truth but to fight for his client. In his office, he advises. Standards of ethics are applicable to his behavior. The ecological point of view proposes rather similar tasks and ethical standards for the psychotherapist. It is fortunate for the legal profession that physiological theory, although partially developed, as we have seen in Plato's *Republic,* was never taken so far as to propose an energy behind justice.

CHAPTER SEVEN

Social Organisms, Networks, and Interfaces: Structure

> The final Buddhist view of the world . . . is not so different from the world view of Western science. . . . Poetically, it is symbolized as a vast network of jewels, like drops of dew upon a multidimensional spider web. Looking closely at any single jewel, one beholds in it the reflections of all the others.
>
> ALLAN WATTS

The first section of this chapter is devoted to a critical assessment of two of the major concepts of social structure postulated by individual psychiatry: individual and environment. After the "delusion" of personal individuality and the idea of the "average expectable environment" are explored, the transfer of these notions to social groups is considered. The adaptive metapsychological point of view is dealt with in the course of this discussion rather than accorded special status in a separate chapter.

Following this criticism of the dualistic conception of individual and environment, the concepts of network and interface are presented as alternative and preferred formulations describing social structure from the standpoint of social psychiatric theory. After different kinds of social aggregations among biological organisms are discussed, the structural characteristics of networks are delineated. One of the most important of these—the social interface—is then illustrated and analyzed at some length. Finally the relevance and application of these concepts to individual and group psychiatric treatment contexts are briefly reviewed.

INDIVIDUAL AND ENVIRONMENT

I. The Delusion of Personal Individuality

The notion of a unique individual mental life is a basic assumption of individual psychiatry and an unacceptable one to social psychiatry; as such, it represents a major controversy between these two viewpoints. The issue actually includes two components: whether or not the individual patient as such constitutes the proper unit of study, and whether each individual personality is unique. Following the pattern established by the clinical or medical model of nineteenth-century medicine, psychiatrists have traditionally thought it feasible to describe and treat a completely independent, discrete entity, the individual patient, whose personality presumably could be influenced in psychotherapy regardless of his physical or social environment. It was further assumed that a patient's personality, like his heart, consisted of universal or species-wide characteristics (e.g., ideas, motives, impulses) so arranged as to constitute a unique constellation. Like other organs, the personality (or mind) came to be thought of as subdermal, existing under the skin, located somewhere within the body.

Harry Stack Sullivan was one of the first psychiatrists to attack the traditional focus on the individual patient as the basis for study and the belief in his uniqueness. In 1944 he gave a lecture entitled, "The Illusion of Personal Individuality," in which he criticized the idea of the uniqueness of the individual and asserted that "we are all more alike than different." Instead of regarding personality as a subdermal entity analogous to the heart or liver, he redefined it as "the relatively enduring pattern of recurrent interpersonal situations which characterize a human life" (1, p. 111). Rather than study the individual patient as an isolated phenomenon, he preferred to focus on the social transactions which the patient characteristically engaged in with people important to him, including the therapist. At the very heart of his theory was the belief that the study of the individual was to be frankly and openly abandoned and that his social relationships and the structure of his social world were to be studied instead. In a commentary on his 1944 lecture, Perry (2) reported that Sullivan did not want to engage in "unrewarding argument," and so did not prepare this paper for publication, although a transcription of the talk was published posthumously (3).

If Sullivan was shy of argument, the same could hardly be said of John Dewey and Arthur Bentley (4). In 1949 they published *Knowing and the Known,* which was remarkable for its support of both of Sullivan's contentions: that the study of the individual should be replaced by a study of his transactions, and that great controversy from many disciplines would be provoked by this assertion. Even their imagery was similar to Sullivan's. Where Sullivan, searching for metaphors, said that the self was interdependent on the environment and could not be separated from it ("A classical instance of this interdependence is the organism's relation to oxygen . . . [3, p. 200]"), Dewey and Bentley wrote: "Organisms do not live without air and water, not without food ingestion and radiation. They live, that is, as much in processes across and 'through' skins as in processes 'within' skins . . . (4, p. 130)." While Sullivan spoke of an illusion of personal individuality, Dewey and Bentley wrote:

> Transactionally viewed, a widening or narrowing of attention is about all that remains indicated by such words as "social" and "individual." . . . if one insists on considering individual and social as different in character, then a derivation of the former from the latter

would, in our judgment, be much simpler and more natural than an attempt to produce a social by joining or otherwise organizing presumptive individuals. In fact most of the talk about the 'individual' is the very finest kind of an illustration of isolation from every form of connection carried to an extreme of absurdity that renders inquiry and intelligent statement impossible (4, p. 142).

The British philosopher Ryle made similar observations. He also rejected the notion of an individual mind and declared: "I shall speak of it, with deliberate abusiveness, as 'the dogma of the Ghost in the Machine.' I hope to prove that it is entirely false, and false not in detail but in principle. It is not merely an assemblage of particular mistakes. It is one big mistake" (5, p. 15).

This brief review should suffice to demonstrate dissatisfaction of a very strong sort with the ideas of an individual psyche and its uniqueness. But this is only one half of the duality. If "individual" is an unacceptable entity, so must be its twin, "environment."

II. The Average Expectable Individual

A basic concept of the adaptive point of view of psychoanalytic theory is Hartmann's notion of an "average expectable environment." He wrote in 1939, "As an indispensable factor in assessing an individual's powers of adaptation we would single out his relation to an 'average expectable environment'" (6, p. 16). Since the introduction of this concept, psychoanalytic and dynamic psychiatry have presumed that the environment is standard while the individual is seen as variable or unique. In other words, it is generally believed that all people face essentially the same situations which some personalities can tolerate and some cannot. Epigrammatically, the social psychiatrist can be seen as making the reverse set of assumptions: he postulates an average expectable individual and sets out to examine the unusual aspects of his environment. (This rephrasing is inaccurate, since it implies acceptance of the underlying duality—individual and environment—which is not actually acknowledged.)

A. The Neurological Underpinnings The continued acceptance by most psychiatrists, following the psychoanalytic tradition, of the notion of the individual psyche seems a function of the essentially neurological assumptions they bring to the task. It must be remembered that Freud began his career as a neurologist and continued to think in such terms even after he turned his attention to psychiatric issues. He later tried to abandon neurological explanation, as he declared in his famous credo in Chapter VII of *The Interpretation of Dreams:* "I shall remain on psychological grounds." If, however, a distinction is maintained between Freud's clinical theory and his general theory or metapsychology, it becomes clear that he remained inconsistent in this area. He himself subsequently noted that, "It is the therapeutic technique alone that is purely psychological; the theory does not by any means fail to point out that neuroses have an organic basis" (7, p. 135). If, for example, conversion hysteria is considered, it can be shown that, in spite of the fact that Freud's psychological study of conversion seems straightforward, the model—the metapsychology—used to organize assumptions about hysteria is neurological. In referring to the "mysterious leap from the mind to the body" underlying hysteria, Freud was thinking in terms of psychic energy converted (hence *conversion* hysteria) in such a way as to travel over actual neurological pathways.

In general, as Holt (8) has documented in detail, Freud continued to use neurological terminology and propositions long after disclaiming such a model. Methodological clarity about the nature and status of the non-neurological theory he said he was building was never attained. Furthermore, he never yielded the underlying assumption that there was a psychic apparatus whose location was the brain, that its pathways were nerve tracts and its energy neurophysiological in nature. Although hysteria was investigated early in Freud's career, the same basic explanation is used thirty years later to explain the physical symptoms of anxiety which Freud went so far as to call the normal prototype of neurologically caused hysteria (9, p. 20). This has sometimes been referred to as "brain mythology." These notions and assumptions have never been explicitly abandoned by psychoanalytic theory, and underlie much of the thinking current today about the subdermal individual psyche.

B. Symptom Choice and Responsibility   The ideas of Sullivan, Dewey, Bentley, and Ryle suggest that a disordered life cannot be explained solely on the basis of individual characteristics or motivations, that it is not helpful to think in terms of individual structural weakness such as an ego deficit to account for behavioral disturbances. Numerous factors and forces deriving from social, physical, and cultural influences as well as genetic predispositions act in complex interaction to produce behavior which is labeled symptomatic; it is no more meaningful to assign all responsibility to the patient, as is implied when one speaks of his "symptom choice," than it is to employ exclusively cultural factors in such an explanation. Furthermore, the report of the patient about his biographical data or his symptoms is of limited utility, since the patient has no privileged access to material about his life. Finally, disordered behavior almost always involves more than one person; it is difficult to conceive of psychopathological behavior occurring in a social vacuum and in fact impossible to label it as such in the absence of a fellow man who assigns the diagnosis. Related to this is the matter of cultural relativism; what may be deemed sick in one culture can be quite acceptable in another. The clinical futility of the individual approach in many situations can be documented by numerous examples from family therapy where the referred patient may be diagnosed as well as the spouse, the children, and the grandparents. When the index patient, for instance a depressed wife, is seen individually, this may inadvertently lead to poor treatment because of a failure to take into account her husband, who has approached her brother in a homosexual fashion; the husband's mother, who shaved him every morning until he was married; the wife's 250-pound mother, who spends most of her life in bed and turned the task of taking care of the wife's brother over to her until she was married; and so forth. Individual diagnosis, even if it takes others into account, leads to an infinite regress of diagnoses extending into the lateral family, neighbors, and employers, and backwards through many generations. For all these reasons, the social context and important people surrounding the person labeled as patient are inextricably implicated in his disturbed behavior to the point where it is meaningless to try to assign responsibility for it to any one source.

The notion that the patient is not solely responsible for his behavior is indirectly supported by the undeniable fact that it is not primarily his behavior but other contingencies that determine the psychiatric diagnosis and treatment received. Whether someone is sent to jail as a criminal, to a church as sinful, to a psychiatrist as sick, or to a welfare agency as indigent depends largely on his social class, geographical location, age, and skin color, and how those about the patient regard and evaluate his behavior (10). Decisions about diagnosis and treatment are thus as much social as medical. In this context, it becomes apparent that it is far more helpful to acknowledge the variability of environments than to emphasize their sameness, and, furthermore, that recognition of the impact of situational variables relieves the patient of part of the responsibility and, therefore, burden, for his problems. In this framework, disturbed behavior is less likely to be regarded as a shameful condition caused by individual weaknesses, and is seen more accurately as the outcome of vastly complex interactions of many factors from different sources. In this sense one can agree with Sarason (11) that "patients come by their problems honestly," instead of thinking of them as less than adequate human beings who have nobody to blame but themselves.

C. The Adaptive Point of View The notion of an average expectable environment seems reasonable enough until it is seriously investigated. Individual behavior varies enormously, but if we think for a moment, so do environments. It would certainly be difficult to argue that any two people have lived in such similar social, cultural, and physical environments that they could be meaningfully "averaged." In fact, it is currently asserted that every family comprises a unique culture which is differently experienced by each member because of variations in age and children's birth order. This approach may be excessively atomistic, but it illustrates the weakness of trying to "average" a multitude of factors which cannot be summed and whose interactions may be as significant as their individual roles.

Rausch, Goodrich, and Campbell (12) have sought a compromise by suggesting that the concept of average expectable environment is relevant to some cultures but not to others. They observe that certain societies, such as the late Victorian era of Freud's day, are so homogeneous that adaptation consists of coping with what *is*, with the universally known and accepted rules of the times. In this context, the idea of average expectable environment is meaningful and relevant. But in other societies such as ours, there are so few generally acknowledged guidelines for behavior that adaptation involves the search for new solutions to new problems, working out what *is to be*. Here Hartmann's concept is less applicable. A major problem with this explanation is its strategy of selective application. Admittedly life is different, and probably easier, in a traditional culture than in a rapidly changing one. But is it helpful to use one psychological explanation for one and not for another? The explanatory power of a theory is surely weakened if it must seek out special cases.

I doubt that Freud would have accepted this compromise explanation or, for that matter, much of the theory of the adaptive point of view. He was certainly aware of the impact of environment on behavior, and dealt with this recognition in two ways. First, he assumed that major social experiences, such as the Oedipus complex, could be transmitted by heredity if the necessary elements were missing from a given environment. Second, on a more basic philosophical level, he made the decision that every scientist is entitled to focus on certain phenomena and exclude others from his consideration, and that he personally wished to study individual psychology rather than environmental influences on behavior.

An example of Freud's rather Lamarckian notion of the hereditary transmission of interpersonal experiences is found in his case history popularly known as that of the "Wolf Man." In his childhood, this patient was threatened by his nurse with castration, yet he came to fear that his father would thus punish him. Freud accounts for the child's misinterpretation by stating that "at this point, the boy had to fit himself into a phylogenetic schema, and he did so, although his personal experiences may not have agreed with it" (13, p. 565). In his summary of the Wolf Man case he wrote:

> I am inclined to take the view that they [such events] are precipitates from the history of human civilization. The Oedipus complex, which comprises a child's relation to its parents, is one of them—is, in fact, the best known member of its class. Wherever experiences fail to fit in with the hereditary schema, they become remodelled in the imagination. . . . We are often able to see the schema triumphing over the experience of the individual, as when in our present case the boy's father became the castrator and the menace to his infantile sexuality in spite of what was in other respects an inverted Oedipus complex [love of father and fear of castration by mother] (13, p. 603).

On a more basic level, Freud explicitly excluded environmental factors from his study of behavior as a matter of strategy: He believed that scientists were entitled to select certain dimensions of a given problem which their training qualified them to study, and concentrate on these, acknowledging that other approaches may also be relevant. In Joseph Wortis' account of his analysis with Freud, he relates that he asked why Freud ignored the role of environmental factors: "When I attempted to define a neurosis as a maladaptation between an individual and his environment, and said one could prevent neurosis by changing the environment, Freud did not disagree but said that was not a doctor's task" (14, p. 25). On another occasion, Wortis reported the following response:

> "There are a lot of things I don't mention in my books," he [Freud] said. "That's the sort of criticism [that he had not discussed the effect of environmental factors on neurosis] I often hear from the Bolsheviki. I can't discuss everything. I don't discuss climate either, though it is certainly important. I should certainly feel better if I were in a better climate. Certainly money troubles contribute to neurosis. Many things do. You might as well criticize a chemist for not writing about physics . . ." (14, p. 56).

Freud's position is perfectly tenable and is in keeping with a long medical tradition. This becomes apparent on consideration of the medical approach to tuberculosis. Until quite recently, the mythology of the physician was based on the so-called germ theory of disease. For practical purposes the physician focused on the tuberculosis bacillus. Yet no physician was actually ignorant of "environmental influences." The "cause" of tuberculosis can be said to be either the bacillus or, from another point of view, poverty and its associated evils: malnutrition, overcrowding, and exposure. A germ theory would postulate a random distribution of tuberculosis throughout the population which is not in fact the case. One may speculate whether ultimate control of the disease will be brought about by an attack on the bacillus, or on social conditions, which, as Freud pointed out, are not within the traditional competencies of the physician.

The germ theory, using a biological model, has not always been the major explanatory concept in the understanding of disease process; it became widely accepted only at the end of the nineteenth century. Before then, miasma theory based on what was essentially a social or community model had dominated medical thinking since Hippocrates. Miasma theory held that poisonous substances rose up from certain geographical areas and were carried by the winds to cause fevers. It assumed that few if any diseases are entirely independent, uniquely caused entities but rather that disease states are interdependent and even interchangeable. While it has been discredited as the general explanation for the spread of infectious diseases, miasma theory offers a *model* and a set of strategies that may be far more valuable than the germ theory for community health and mental health workers. While it was still accepted, miasma theory led to an emphasis on primary prevention rather than treatment or rehabilitation, an emphasis on the total community and recognition of the need to work with and through community agencies to change overall health patterns. These principles worked well in the past; as Bloom (15) observed, "Miasma theory and the practical programs which it generated have probably done more to raise the general level of health in the world than have programs instituted as a consequence of germ theory" (p. 338). Strategies based on the miasma model seem of continued value at present in the context of social psychiatry.

Because the physician (including the psychiatrist) has not been trained to deal with them, environmental conditions are typically excluded from his plan of attack on a given problem, although he is not oblivious to their impact. This sort of exclusion represents a method for reducing a given problem to manageable size. Thus Freud did not assert an "average expectable environment," but declared instead that he was powerless to influence political, social, architectural, climatic, and economic conditions. It becomes a legitimate question to consider who, indeed, *shall* accept responsibility for changing the environment to promote physical and mental health if physicians and psychiatrists do not feel it is within their competence to do so. As large-scale social planning becomes a growing reality, we may hope that the germ theory explanation of disease and maladjustment will become only one aspect of a broader conceptualization of promoting conditions of health. This will come about not by thinking in terms of average environments but by acknowledging their selective and specific characteristics as they influence human behavior.

In short, the adaptive model starts out by limiting the number of changing or changeable variables that are presumed to influence behavior, and ends up by eliminating from consideration all those environmental characteristics over which psychoanalysts presume they have no control. Like the germ theory, the adaptive model is reductionist in that it simplifies complex issues, and it also blocks relevant paths of inquiry. The adaptive model masks environmental differences, just as the social psychiatric model tends to mask individual differences; both models would be more effective if confined to their specific areas of competence and relevance.

III. The Social Skin: Critique of the Organismic Approach

As the limitations of individual psychiatry become more apparent, it has become fairly common for its metaphors and models to be transferred, largely unaltered, from individuals to groups. This tendency to postulate social organisms possessing the same characteristics formerly attributed to the individual represents a kind of fallacy in which the individual skin is simply extended to include others and so becomes a "social skin." Thus one now hears about the "schizophrenic family" instead of the schizophrenic individual, of the family and its environment instead of the individual and his environment. These are at best misleading formulations, since they imply an awareness of social processes that is not actually present.

The notion of social organisms analogous to individual organisms has long existed in literary contexts. Thus one can find in the Oxford English Dictionary the following entries:

gaggle of geese	shrewdness of apes
pride of lions	crash of rhinos
kindle of kittens	exaltation of larks
cowardice of curs	murmuration of starlings
murder of crows	sedge of herons
pace of asses	walk of snipe
trip of seals	bale of turtles
lepe of leopards	hovel of trout
rafter of turkeys	drift of hogs
sloth of bears	gam of whales
labor of moles	smack of jellyfish

The need to create such "organisms" is also expressed in humor: It is said that three poets tried to find a collective name for three prostitutes walking by. One suggested "a bevy of broads," another "a trey of tarts," and the third "a flourish of strumpets." It is understandable that social organisms are created in such numbers when our tools for thinking about events come from the framework of individual psychiatry.

Once we have given a specific name to a social group (a walk of snipe, a family, a catchment area), it appears to possess collective qualities and an organismic identity which take on a misleading reality. Sussman (16, p. 72) has suggested that the concept of "nuclear family" is a figment of Marriage and the Family courses in college, together with theoretical work. The same phenomenon can be seen when we apply a label to an individual; the conceptual fiction quickly becomes obscured and the named entity seems increasingly real and self-evident. An excellent example of this process is seen in psychiatric diagnosis. Both the old and new American Psychiatric Association Diagnostic Manuals (17) list a long series of diagnostic labels that presumably refer to specific disease entities differing in terms of etiology, disease course, recommended treatment, and eventual outcome. This diagnostic system is based on the precepts of individual psychiatry, uses the biological or medical model of disease, and has raised the status of diagnosis in the mental health professions. Its basic assumptions have yet to be verified, however; no one has been able to demonstrate unique causes for different psychiatric diseases, much less mutually exclusive courses and outcomes. When scrutinized closely, the entities do not seem altogether cohesive or logical, and their defining characteristics lose specificity. For example, the passive-dependent type of personality trait disorder is a "reality" in the official psychiatric nomenclature. It is said to be characterized by "helplessness, indecisiveness, and a tendency to cling to others as a dependent child to a supporting parent" (17, p. 57). On reflection, everyone would agree that there have been times when their behavior must have appeared helpless, clinging, and so forth. The real issues are with whom, where, and how much of the time such behavior is manifested. This leads to a variety of questions about one's setting, about the situation, about the cultural rules and expectations. These may be of little interest in the framework of individual psychiatry, but they are the major issues of social psychiatry.

From the point of view of social psychiatry, these elaborate diagnostic distinctions and differentiations are seen as primarily conceptual fictions. A distinct counterposition is presented: that psychiatric difficulties are to be conceptualized within a single continuum of adaptation or adjustment to the context; as "personal, social and ethical problems in living," according to Szasz (18, p. 295); a disruption of one's "vital balance," as Menninger (19) says; or as a "social breakdown syndrome," following Gruenberg (20). Once the framework of individual psychiatry is rejected, there remains in the traditional format only one diagnosis: "situational maladjustment" and its "stages."

In general, then, it seems apparent that if you believe in a discrete social entity or organism, you are affected by this belief just as you are affected by a diagnostic label. If labels are transferred from individuals to groups while the point of view of individual psychiatry is maintained, little has been achieved. It is not enough to say that we reject the individual psyche but accept the group psyche, reject the individual unconscious but believe in the family unconscious. Our goal must be to discuss social structure without recourse to the individual-environment dichotomous model of individual psychiatry—to develop a model without a skin. As the above-mentioned poets were talking about "flourishes of strumpets," the prostitutes were wondering what to call the social organism they saw before them. One said, "Why not call them a pack of poets"; another said, "How about a run of rhymers"; the third suggested, "A changing of the bards."

NETWORKS

An alternative approach to the analysis of social structures can be found in the social psychiatric concept of *network*. Instead of sharply differentiating figure and ground in a static dichotomy like that of individual and environment, the concept of network consists of interwoven patterns of relationships and events which have no boundaries and encompass all of a given domain, including the observer. A network can include any kind of biological grouping, animal or human, and may involve more than one species if such relationships prevail in the population being described. Although networks are theoretically open-ended and unbounded, they are generally limited for practical purposes in terms of a specific problem of interest to the investigator. (It would be proper, but clumsy, to indicate that when we speak of a network, we really are referring to part of the universal network.)

A network is a field of points, some or all of which are connected to each other. Each point represents both a stimulus for other points and a respondent to the other points. They can be classified in terms of biological types: taxic, biotaxic, and sociotaxic. *Taxis* refers to inanimate stimuli such as geographical or architectural configurations, weather conditions, objects, or things. For instance, an oasis constitutes a stimulus for a fairly permanent gathering of people, and would be represented by a central point in a network describing a population of this sort. *Biotaxis* refers to animate stimuli, such as a person or an animal. *Sociotaxis* refers to social stimuli, which are, in effect, all groups perceived as having a "social skin," such as a family, a political party, or a school class. Rat colonies, for instance, develop a distinctive odor and attack those rats that do not possess it.

Connecting lines between points represent reciprocal interaction. They are drawn in a network if the interactions between the two points are recurrent and meaningful to at least one of those involved (a relationship). The field of points may grow and change, with some being added and others dropping out over a period of time. For example, if one family feuds with another, a line is drawn between the two points representing Family One and Family Two. If the feud becomes sufficiently established it can itself become a stimulus for others, such as a group of worried neighbors, and therefore the feud becomes a point in the network. The feud can also be resolved, like that between the Montagues and Capulets, and thus disappear from the network.

Examination of connecting lines in a particular area of the network will reveal a certain kind of mesh or knit which may be either loose or tight. Bott (21) has suggested that connectedness or involvement has certain limits: If one is tightly connected with one part of a network, it is not possible to be also very involved with other parts. This makes sense in terms of the limits inevitably experienced: If one is extremely involved at work, there is less time for the family; if one is enormously devoted to one's parents, there is less time for friends; and so forth. Such limits can be emotional, temporal, or spatial.

We can observe other characteristics of a network besides its mesh. In some of its areas different types of stimuli may be more prominent and active. Comparing Japan and the United States, it can be observed that sociotaxic stimuli such as family or religion are more important to the Japanese than biotaxic stimuli (individual people), while the converse is probably true in the United States. Accordingly, the nature of the fabric in each society will vary in terms of its knit in the terms of the percentage of nodal points which are sociotaxic. In a primitive society, many of the nodal points might be other species and inanimate objects.

Use of the network model facilitates a redefinition of personality in terms of behavioral transactions rather than the subdermal psyche of individual psychiatry. A personality can be described as a view of a network seen as the connections radiating from a selected point. Whenever one point of a network is singled out as a focus, one is describing the personality of that point. Accordingly, to paraphrase Sullivan, personality is the relatively enduring pattern of recurrent situations which revolve around a specific point in the network. In this definition anything that is a stimulus, a point, can have a personality. Dogs, families, things, and places can be meaningfully described in this way. This definition of personality goes only slightly further theoretically than Sullivan's by its inclusion of inanimate and social stimuli. These implications have generally been neglected but are indicated nevertheless in Sullivan's thinking: namely, that large numbers of people, things, and ideas are involved in a personality and must be considered in a treatment plan. To speak of "the relatively enduring pattern of recurrent interpersonal situations" would include, for example, all the people who could or would come to a person's funeral (admittedly a lugubrious thought, but remember they come to mourn, i.e., with due purpose). If one's dog remains by one's grave, as the romantic stories would have it, we must include the dog in the network. Since people have been known to die rather than sacrifice their property, these material goods become significant components in their descriptions. Such entities are included, not because they are believed to have personalities in a supernatural sense, but because they exercise a significant influence on the behavior of the person or persons being described.

In short, the object of this discussion is to demonstrate the utility of the network model to replace the rather ineffective efforts to isolate and describe with precision the individual personality. As noted, the network model is designed to include factors that extend any number of "generations" away. Although for practical reasons boundaries are established for a given network, far more data is included than is usually the case in studies of individuals. Particularly in situations where behavior looks peculiar, it is profitable to keep extending the boundaries of inquiry, the skin, until some sense is made out of the situation. There are already individuals experimenting with the treatment of natural groups in a network with as many as seventy members (22). The network concept can lead to treatment of such large groups by a logical extension of theory: when a pattern is delineated, it becomes artificial to ignore "second-generation" effects where one person influences another through a third, fourth, or fifth. For example, grandfather can unwittingly influence grandchild (to be lazy, timid, etc.) through his relationship with mother.

Use of the network model entails certain problems in obtaining relevant data and organizing it so that it is useful. Although this chapter is meant to explore the theoretical approach rather than practical difficulties, it may be useful to note in passing some of the more obvious hazards. First, patients tend to come to therapy sharing the prevailing assumptions of their therapists. Accordingly, their biographical musings often focus on the nursery years and exclude current friends and relatives. Such patients can be taught to provide the kind of information usually reserved for anthropological studies, such as floor plans of their home, description of a typical day, and so forth. Organizing data about social transactions is also a rather novel task, but solutions have been suggested in the literature on animal behavior, such as Southwick's (23) studies of primate groups.

As we have noted, a network resembles a fishnet. There are nodal points and connecting lines, and these may be bunched and grouped unevenly depending on the extent of impact of the various stimuli or points. There is also another dimension or quality to this model that has not yet been mentioned: the spaces between. When a large network is observed and its points are delineated, there can occur a figure-ground reversal in which the large "holes" in the fabric begin to take on more interest than the designs (personalities) woven in it. These spaces are here called "interfaces."

INTERFACES

At a recent national conference on community psychiatry it was suggested that "the most pressing need is to develop conceptual models and theories to form an orderly development of practice" (24, p. 175). One model that is available from the observations of anthropologists, political scientists, and psychiatrists as they study the effects of reaching the boundaries of sociocultural systems is that of network interface. After a brief discussion of the notion of an interface in a network, I shall discuss various dynamics at interfaces from an individual and a group point of view. Following this, I shall offer some brief comments on the structural aspects of interfaces and the relevance of the concept to treatment strategies.

I. Interface: The Model

As many housewives know, an interface can be a third piece of cloth between two others. In dress patterns the term refers to a separate piece of cloth, unseen because it is sewn between others to reinforce or stiffen. Precisely because the word can be used for the separate piece of cloth and not for the side or face that is in contact with another, the person unfamiliar with the term finds he knows nothing in the social sciences to which he might apply it. It suggests a new ingredient in the environment of the social sciences. This points up the fact that social organizations have always been seen as nesting within other social groups (e.g., families *in* cultures) and never in some sort of neutral "ground substance" or background. In the social sciences, the search for answers has always gone on in terms of the intercellular pathology, so to speak. It can thus be said that the social sciences have not used the concept of *space*. Although today we take space, empty space, for granted, this was not always the case. Descartes, for example, did not; he had to assume that every "space" was occupied. This presents problems, since any dimension, such as a cubic inch, can be further divided into smaller units which must also be occupied. In any event, we now think of the atom as mostly emptiness.

The cellular analogy mentioned above is worth pursuing further. Pathologists previously examined a very similar hierarchical series of structures (cell components *in* the cell *in* the organ component *in* the organ and so forth). However, when they were led by Klemperer to look outside the cell itself into the surrounding ground substance, they found a series of disorders—rheumatoid arthritis, for instance—which were profitably thought of as residing, not in the cell, but in the supporting ground substance itself, the *space* around the cell. Similarly, social systems have never been presumed to be surrounded by a neutral matrix; there were nothing but individuals within ever-increasing concentric circles of social systems. It is for this reason that *interface* is such an instructive word. It clearly implies that a model of social systems embedded in something that is not a social system *can* be profitably examined. What emerges in conjunction with the network concept is that this embedding matrix can be conceived of as having both dimensions and processes of its own.

II. Interface Dynamics

In this section six dynamics that occur in the interfaces of social systems are discussed. In the interests of brevity and the development of an overall perspective, descriptions and illustrations are kept to a minimum. They include: A) interface ("culture") shock; B) interface penetration ("snuggling"); C) Induction ("acculturation," "crossover," "family suction"); D) resonance ("mirroring," "psychosocial replication"); E) interface stationing ("tourist-native transaction"); and F) interface accentuation ("the ugly American").

A. **Interface shock**   The best-known examples of difficulty at an interface stem from anthropological reports about the occasional severe discomfort of individuals in foreign cultures. Although it has been of some personal concern to anthropologists for many years as a sort of occupational hazard, and of current interest to the Peace Corps, which has studied it at some length (25), Oberg (26) was the first to stress the importance of the phenomenon. As the result of experience with Americans working in Brazil on a joint project he observed:

> Culture shock is precipitated by the anxiety that results from losing all one's familiar cues. These cues include the thousand and one ways in which we orient ourselves to the situations of daily life: when to shake hands and what to say when we meet people, make purchases, when to accept and when to refuse invitations, when to take statements seriously and when not. Those cues to behavior (which may be words, gestures, facial expressions or customs) are acquired in the course of growing up and are as much a part of our culture as the language we speak. All of us depend for our peace of mind and our efficiency on hundreds of cues, most of which we do not carry on a level of conscious awareness (26).

Two points can be added to Oberg's comments. First, the phenomenon under discussion occurs in situations besides the movement of individuals from one culture to another. One can observe similar shock when two people from very different backgrounds get married (27). It can also be seen in schools where the teachers and pupils are very dissimilar culturally, as in most slums. The phenomenon therefore seems to be generic and the more general label *interface shock* is suggested in place of *culture shock*. A second point is that Oberg's description emphasizes too exclusively postural-kinetic codes as the source of the problem. While this is true, it is incomplete; we all depend for our comfort on a familiar network of people, things, ideas, and conventions. Their absence induces tension. It is essentially an isolation experience, including isolation from postural-kinetic codes, but also from other stimuli as well. When experiencing interface shock, the individual can be seen as occupying the empty space between cultural networks.

B. Interface Penetration   Under the inelegant term *snuggling*, interface penetration is another concept to come from informal anthropological self-observation, and refers to situations of wide cultural disparity. It is exemplified by the American who on visiting Japan suddenly and quite immediately becomes what he thinks of as Japanese. He is, of course, a gross caricature of the

Japanese, but it is said that he has "snuggled." A young nurse cited by Arnold (25) as a case of culture shock because she shunned her American co-volunteers and associated exclusively with local residents can be seen as a snuggler.

Snuggling, like interface shock, can be observed within a culture. The newcomer to the staff of a treatment center who appears to have gobbled up whole the dominant ideology (whether psychoanalysis or social psychiatry) is snuggling. He is usually rewarded in a fashion, but his grasp of the actual details is not anywhere near as good as it appears. He is not a stable or dependable member of the group, so that this sort of penetration of the interface resembles an infection which under stress or in sufficient numbers will seriously weaken the network.

On the level of the family, individuals who have hidden their family origins, perhaps to facilitate their upward mobility, are extremely susceptible to snuggling. A peripheral position in one's own network is, perhaps, a function of the mechanism of snuggling. Whereas interface shock is thought of as being lost in empty space between networks, snuggling (interface penetration) can be compared to a first-stage landing on a foreign planet. From clinical observation, "going native" in the sense used here is more like an invasion from outer space—that is, of potential danger to the "host" network.

C. Induction   Whether acculturation or induction into a system can be accomplished in one generation is an issue that must be decided by anthropologists. Analogous processes that appear in family therapy are known as "going under" or "family suction" (28): an outsider is drawn into the family's system and his behavior begins to resemble that of the family members although this is not his intention. The process of induction is one of the hazards of family therapy, since the therapist cannot change the family system and rules of conduct unless he remains on the outside, able to function autonomously. From the standpoint of family therapy, countertransference is a special case of this phenomenon.

D. Resonance   Systems in contact tend to resemble each other; there is a resonance between them like that between two tuning forks. Block (29) has spoken of psychosocial replication in which particular family systems are replicated in residential treatment centers by the staff members. On a different level, class or economic systems can replicate themselves in the institutions with which they come in contact. For example, there is a tendency to "think poor" among schoolteachers who have spent some time in ghetto schools. One assistant principal found it difficult to realize that he had the same funds to buy the same books that were being used by schools in the better part of town. The parents had assumed that their schools must be poor, and this became mirrored within the school administration. Across the gap between the networks was some process that tended to create a resonance.

E. Interface Stationing   The tourist and the native evidently enjoy their location at the interface. (In the fashion I am using these terms, *tourist* must be distinguished from *traveler,* and *native* from *resident.*) There are individuals in every system who enjoy sightseeing, and others who like quaint costumes and the profit that can be gained by allowing themselves to become involved with tourists. This is not necessarily a phenomenon of backward countries; in Belgium there are costumed women who station themselves along major tourist routes and make lace on the sidewalk, demanding payment to be photographed. Within a given culture, a comparable phenomenon is that of slumming or visiting ethnically unique areas.

Intergenerational conflicts today often take the form of interface stationing. Adolescents who call themselves beatniks, hippies, free men, or just teenagers increase their visibility to the older generation, which enjoys or at least responds vigorously to their activities. It is inaccurate to acknowledge only one side of such equations since both are necessary for the phenomenon to exist. Thus the Haight-Ashbury district of San Francisco was an area where hippies paraded the streets in bizarre costumes while busloads of older toursists came just to look at them. From this perspective, the tourists are just as involved as the natives.

F. Interface Accentuation   This type of interface behavior frequently depends on irritation. Finding himself at an interface, the individual suddenly becomes more like his system of origin, very often in just those situations that are particularly irksome to members of the other groups. The Jew who decides to follow dietary rituals for the first time in his life upon moving from Brook-

lyn to Kansas exemplifies such behavior. A more topical example
is provided by the American Negroes who have recently taken to
letting their hair grow long and wearing *dashikes* and other African attire; since these sartorial fashions are most popular among
black militant and nationalist groups, their purpose of accentuat-
ing differences is underlined. Milder examples would include the
Puerto Rican who suddenly cannot speak English in a clinic, or
the ethnic seating arrangements at Parents' Association and Head
Start parents' meetings.

III. Interface Dynamics From the Point of View of the Group

Meier (30) has noted that when two cultural streams come
into extended contact, there are five possible outcomes:
A. Dissolution of one culture (the "vanishing Bushman")
B. Communalization (ghetto formation, slavery)
C. Conflict
D. Assimilation (the melting pot)
E. Selective combination (hybrid vigor)

A. Dissolution Anthropologists have described several cultural
groups that visibly faded out following their subjugation by other
groups. Linton (31, p. 137) observed, when he visited the
Marquesans in the 1920's after a prolonged period of overt conflict with Western colonizers, that "they adopted the only means
of dignified and effective resistance which was open to them, they
ceased to breed. This was a perfectly deliberate measure, the people preferring extinction to subjugation." However "deliberate"
such measures were, from today's perspective, one can only wish
that Linton had chosen to study this process in detail in addition
to producing his masterful reconstruction of the original Marquesan culture. How is such a decision made? Through what processes does an entire population cooperate with it? The issue becomes even more complex when we consider reports of biologists,
also studying population interfaces, that animal groups as varied
as mice and elephants also "cease to breed" under certain demo-
graphic conditions such as overcrowding.

B. Communalization Studies of ghetto formation and their relationship to other forms of communalization such as the "wandering bands of Romany" are urgently needed today. While some investigators have noted the positive attributes of distinct ethnic communities within a larger population in terms of facilitating the tasks of transition for newly migrating groups, the drawbacks are far more obvious.

C. Conflict One hardly needs to search intensively to find evidence of conflict as a result of contact between disparate social systems. One can think of dissolution, communalization, or assimilation as various outcomes following a more or less prolonged era of confrontation between minority and dominant social groups. The sort of conflict conceived here is a more stable condition, arising when the minority group is no longer willing to accept inferior status. Something of this sort seems to be emerging in the American Negro community at the present time. It is perhaps ironic that acknowledgment by the majority group of the minority's deprivations can exacerbate relations between them.

D. Assimilation Known as "the melting pot," assimilation has long been regarded as an ideal solution to problems of group differences in the United States. Whether cultural and value conflicts are ever resolved in terms of the transformation of one group *into* the other is a moot point today. Even if this process was relevant in the past, it is today questionable whether the "receiving" society is large enough numerically to absorb those who are presently not assimilated. It is also debatable whether all deviant social groups would wish to become absorbed in this manner.

E. Selective Combination Meier (30) has suggested the concept of hybrid vigor to explain the nature of Puerto Rican character, which presumably includes both Indian and Spanish qualities. Other examples of selective combination include English society after the Norman invasion, the prominent use of words of Jewish origin in the United States, and the recent wide adoption of Negro slang.

It remains to be seen how valuable these concepts will be when applied to the area of social and community psychiatry. One obvious limitation of Meier's classification is that it does not simultaneously take into account both of the cultures involved, but focuses solely on the behavior of the minority group. It is unclear what characteristics of the dominant culture influence the choice of outcome, or whether such considerations are always relevant. Such issues might profitably be rephrased in terms of the interface model.

A good example of the need to consider both sides of the situation, both groups in contact, is the police-Negro ghetto situation. One source, for instance, gives a graphic presentation which attends to only one side of the interface and therefore is ultimately inaccurate:

> The ghetto atmosphere was illuminated last week in a study prepared for the President's Commission on Law Enforcement. In a survey of three cities—Chicago, Washington, and Boston—the study found that four out of every five white policemen working in Negro neighborhoods have prejudiced attitudes toward Negroes. The report estimated that 45% of the white police (and, surprisingly, nearly 10% of the Negro police) showed near pathological hostility. . . . Though the survey found that police are rarely "unprofessional" in their contacts with Negroes, the conclusion was inescapable that this antipathy is felt by ghetto dwellers . . . (32).

What such a survey does not reveal is the Negroes' "near pathological" attitudes toward the police. Mattick, working with lower-class Negro nursery school children, noted: ". . . when mother did not open the door at the first knock, she was assumed to be 'dead,' or 'in de hospital,' or *in jail*. Equally a baby brother with a minor illness was expected to get worse; 'He die and de *cops* take 'em' " (33, p. 683; italics mine). The futility of assigning the responsibility for this conflict to only one of these groups has been emphasized in other studies of difficult situations between social systems such as parts of a family. Equally pointless is the attempt to decide who started the conflict (34). It is probably more practical to approach the police-ghetto problem from the point of view of pathological dynamics at the interface than to imply, as in the commission report, that the police or individual policemen are hosts to a pathological antipathy. This survey, it must be noted, states that policemen are rarely unprofessional in their conduct. In this case, a much more intangible quality of the situation must be the focus of attention.

IV. Treatment Strategies

Although it is usually assumed that psychotherapy occurs between an individual patient and an individual therapist, each can be seen as the representative of a separate social system. On a broader plane of generalization, each can be regarded as being at an interface between their social systems. Recent work in the observation and treatment of social networks indicates that the therapist must frequently compete with many "outsiders" who comment on or otherwise influence the process. This has sometimes been expressed in terms of their being many "eidetic individuals" in the consultation room. Perceptive psychotherapists like Clara Thompson were aware of certain patterns of discussion outside of analysis; for instance, if the analyst is male, a female acquaintance is often involved in corroborating, amplifying, or otherwise modifying his influence (35). Speck, one of the most active and inventive in examining this "absent member" phenomenon, has vividly illustrated the point: "In yet another case a brother-in-law paid for the family treatment with the proviso that the family would come and discuss what happened in each session with him, and he reserved the right to tell the family what to accept from the therapist and what not to accept" (36, p. 209). Such observations make more understandable the traditional psychoanalytic principle of accepting only those patients for psychoanalysis who finance their treatment out of capital and not earnings or borrowed money (37, p. 32).

A word might be said about the "illusion of the individual therapist." Therapists belong to social networks in the same way that patients do. Like the patient, the therapist can be thought of as stationing himself at the interface of his social system. The involvement of the therapist in a social network can also be illustrated by considering the splinter groups within the psychoanalytic movement. If it is indeed true that systems in contact, such as families and psychotherapeutic networks, exert strong pulls on each other in which one is likely to triumph over the other in some fashion, it is understandable that local groups of therapists would tend to form tight units in self-defense. Schisms (or inter-faces) with other tightly knit therapeutic groups would then be an unfortunate side-effect of the cohesion necessary to protect members from being inducted or crossing over into other social systems.

In short, it seems increasingly evident that psychotherapy is not done by one individual to another, but goes on between social systems. Recognition of this notion leads to certain treatment strategies. For example, at a residential treatment center, certain interface dynamics might be anticipated between the social net-work of the staff and that of the patient population. To render these inevitable interactions therapeutically constructive, one might try to achieve a tightly organized pattern of staff behavior resembling that desired among the patients. If this staff behavior was consistently maintained by all members, there would be less inclination for staff members to drift into other patterns, and at the same time there would be a pull on the patients to mirror the staff behavior. By viewing the staff system itself as the treatment vehicle and obtaining enough time to have consultants deal with it and its interactions with the patient system (the interface), it would be possible to establish a staff system that would be able to quickly repair the effects of pulls exerted on it by the patient pop-ulation. By the very nature of this approach it is assumed that when patients are discharged into their home community, they will be inclined to adopt other behaviors. It would then seem that residential treatment alone is not adequate, but that some sort of follow-up approach must be designed as a subsequent stage of treatment. Accordingly, organization of the treatment center as a "halfway house" with considerable family and commu-nity contact becomes a preferred treatment strategy.

The details of treatment strategies for each of the interface dy-namics discussed have just begun to be explored. It would be be-yond the scope of this chapter to discuss them in detail. To a lim-ited degree, awareness of these dynamics is in itself helpful. A clearer understanding of the tasks that follow this awareness is more helpful. Snuggling, for example, can be curtailed by an open acknowledgment and exposure of one's system of origin and encouragement of enlightened criticism of the system that is penetrated. Because both sides of the interface must be consid-ered, there are tasks to be achieved by both the snuggler and the system that is penetrated, and even for members of the snuggler's original social system or "system of origin." In the case of a snuggler then, factors beyond the individual are considered which can lead to considerable environmental manipulation. Another treatment strategy concerns influencing the amount of distance between social systems. While such distance cannot be directly measured, it can be increased or decreased. This can represent a major strategy in treating groups. When such distances are reduced, for instance when a group of middle-class teachers observes a lower-class family (or vice versa), many of the processes (shock, snuggling, etc.) may appear and can then be dealt with therapeutically. In summary, the interface model is intended to expedite both the description and treatment of social systems and their behavior in relation to other social and environmental stimuli.

CONCLUSION

By the very nature of the theory proposed here it must follow that a new structural model as well as the complete new metapsychological model proposed in this book will suffer the fates described above when two sociocultural streams or networks meet at an interface. It may shock, develop fickle friends who snuggle toward it, and encourage needless accentuation of differences. How to manage such responses, in the case of the model presented here and in the sample situations presented in the text, must be the concern of everybody. While new approaches are called for, they are also reacted to in specific fashions that sometimes unwittingly defeat them, even by the very people who have pleaded for their presentation.

CHAPTER EIGHT

The Healing
Fictions:
Pathogenesis

He is now confronted with the necessity of con-
veying to his patients the healing fiction, the meaning that quickens—for it is this that the patient
longs for, over and above all that reason and
science can give him. The patient is looking for
something that will take possession of him and
give meaning and form to the confusion of his
neurotic mind.

C. G. JUNG

Government agencies have become increas-
ingly interested in evaluating the quality of medical services as
they assume a larger share of their cost. Although various medical
societies claim that they adequately regulate standards of competence, the government's interest in such control is plausible for
several reasons. If an international comparison is made of various
health statistics such as infant mortality, the United States does
not head the list. Approaching assessment from another route, it
has been found that professors of medicine who observe general

practitioners judge most of them to be deficient in some way. If some less direct index of medical quality such as a doctor's record system is observed, it is found that 40 percent of such records are illegible. Finally, if patients are asked directly whether they are satisfied with treatment received, many report that they are not, as a recent crop of books testifies. In short, as any good administrator knows, an impartial quality-control system is necessary. This is recognized within medicine itself. Since perfection is the only acceptable standard, it is understandable that many physicians claim that they would not send their own relatives to 60 percent of the medical profession. With such an interest in quality and costs of a stated product—medical treatment—we are faced with the problem of governmental regulation of medicine and the future task of efficient bureaucratic medicine.

BUREAUCRATIC VERSUS SOCIALIZED MEDICINE

The Armed Services and the Veterans Administration, seldom regarded as bastions of socialism, have bureaucratic medicine already. So do most countries that refer to their medicine as socialized. How socialism got involved in the issue of bureaucratic medicine, particularly among knowledgeable commentators, is puzzling. It is, in fact, an error. That the state pays the medical bills is merely a bureaucratic fact. Issues of medical cost and quality are neither socialistic nor capitalistic. Questions such as "why must we pay?" "Why do the rich have better treatment?" "Why can't medicine be free like the police or the school system?" are not very radical questions and in addition overlook the enormous popular dissatisfaction with these paradigmatic systems themselves. These questions take exception not to the industry or the product but only to the fee for service. Common as this approach may be among so-called socialist critics of medicine, it represents inadequate social theory. The purpose of this chapter is to show that questions about the product itself, i.e., current medical practice, including the treatment of mental as well as physical disease, are currently in order.

To understand the full implications of the task, one must first recognize that associated with contemporary medicine of the body or mind is a considerable amount of ideology intimately related to the structure of our society. When the average man goes to the average physician, he goes to an allopath. With decreasing probability he might also go to an osteopath, homeopath, or chiropractor. The general public does not realize that there are several separate and distinct schools of medicine, although state governments have had to deal with the problem in terms of licensing procedures. In New York State, for example, chiropractors are licensed; their area of professed competence overlaps that of the M.D. In some California hospitals, admissions go alternately to the osteopathic service, where physicians call themselves D.O.'s and the allopathic service, where physicians are M.D.'s. With choice of healer one thus chooses a school or ideology of medicine. Although most people regard medicine as a compendium, a sort of grab-bag of useful techniques that have been assembled over the years by practical men, it is also a philosophy, a way of life or school of thought. Further, the patient is often inducted into a particular school just as his doctor has been. While most of us do not feel that we have been programmed to respond in any given way, we characteristically formulate feelings of illness in allopathic terms.

Evidence supporting the notion of medical ideologies come from two sources: cross-cultural research and studies of those patients who decide to visit their doctors because of basically nonmedical problems. It has long been observed that other cultures do not necessarily formulate their complaints as we do. An American urban doctor is at a loss when faced with "the miseries" in Appalachia or *empacho* in Puerto Rico. Such problems as suicide, which loom large in our society, seem absurd to the Hopi, among whom it does not occur. Following the second approach, it has been asserted for several hundred years by various analysts of patient populations that roughly 60 percent of those who consult a general practitioner, whether under socialized medicine or not, are not "really" sick. They generally do, however, receive medical treatment; for a while, a blue vitamin B12 injection was a favorite remedy. Such an injection is magic, comparable to the Puerto Rican spiritualist's treatment of *empacho* with the sign of the cross. In view of our interest in bureaucratic problems it is worth noting that it is also expensive magic.

It must not be assumed that doctors go out and solicit fools for

B12 injections. There is no need to invoke the image of a medical conspiracy running a con game on a massive scale. In fact, nothing is less helpful in understanding the problem. We must try to understand the magnetism, the suction that brings together the perplexed patient and the puzzled doctor who both sincerely believe in the efficacy of what they are doing. The doctor is as much a member of the social system as the patient, and both are similarly influenced by it.

It is this 60 percent of the patients in a general practitioner's office appearing for largely non-medical reasons which must represent the focus of any medical reform, not the fee-for-service issue, which is the bureaucratic problem. No solution to the problem of adequate medical care can occur without a prior understanding of the processes that bring such patients and doctors together. As I shall attempt to show here, the problem of grasping and solving the doctors' dilemma requires awareness of the error inherent in the underlying individual psychology model which they use to explain what is happening. From the point of view of social psychiatry, a new perspective becomes available which allows this unresolved and ancient problem to be approached constructively.

THE PLACEBO

Perhaps the hallmark of all forms of medical treatment is the use of drugs. As Sir William Osler has quipped, "The desire to take a medicine is one feature which distinguishes man, the animal, from his fellow creatures" (1). A placebo drug is one that is given more to please than to benefit the patient. *Placebo* is the Latin term for "I shall please"; an alternative definition is "dummy tablet." The "placebo effect," in which this dummy tablet apparently induces medical or psychiatric improvement, is a major puzzle in medicine. Were it a limited observation, an occasional occurrence, the puzzle might be intriguing but unimportant. However, until 1900 or so, placebos were virtually all medicine had to offer and constituted most of the pharmaceutical repertoire of physicians. In more recent times, studies have suggested that somewhere between one-third and two-fifths of all prescriptions are purely placebos (2), so that surely the phenomenon cannot be dismissed as occasional or limited. The function and uses of placebos must be understood before attempting to establish government support for medical treatment. Contributing to the mystery is the curtain of silence about the placebo effect. Dubois (3) reports, "although placebos are scarcely mentioned in the literature, they are administered more than any other group of drugs. . . . Although few doctors admit that they give placebos, there is a placebo ingredient in practically every prescription."

The difficulties in attaining a clear understanding of placebos have two origins. The first concerns the reluctance of physicians to examine their practices from a vantage point outside of their own ideology. The second is that the explanations offered invariably return to inner-space or psychological notions which are unilluminating. To report that placebos work because of a "mental" effect or factor does not explain anything, but simply replaces one mystery with another. Prior to the "mental factor" explanation, the idea of faith healing was invoked to account for the effect produced by pharmaceutically worthless drugs. In the 1500's Paracelsus observed: "Faith in the gods or in the saints cures one, faith in little pills another, hypnotic suggestion a third, faith in a plain common doctor a fourth. . . . Faith in us, faith in our drugs and methods, is the great stock in trade of the profession . . . while we doctors often overlook or are ignorant of our own faith-cures, we are just a wee bit too sensitive about those performed outside our ranks" (2).

Over the course of time, the two most common methods of dealing with the placebo phenomenon have been either exploitation of the placebo effect ("You should treat as many patients as possible with the new drugs while they still have the power to heal" [2]), or an overall rejection of drugs. Thus Oliver Wendell Holmes said in 1860 that most drugs should be thrown "into the sea where it would be better for mankind, and all the worse for the fishes" (4).

Neither physicians nor laymen usually recognize the historical or contemporary limitations of pharmacology. None of the drugs listed by Hippocrates were demonstrably useful, and in fact the first drug to be associated with a specific function was quinine, which Sydenham in the 1600's showed to cure malaria. The contemporary dose of morphine is reportedly 50 to 100 percent greater than that needed to give maximum pain relief (2, p. 131). Many commentators feel that future physicians shall look back at our polypharmacy in the same way we now look upon examples of therapeutics in other ages. For instance, the treatment of Charles II was reported as follows:

> A pint of blood was extracted from his right arm, and a half-pint from his left shoulder, followed by an emetic, two physics, and an enema comprising fifteen substances; the royal head was then shaved and a blister raised; then a sneezing powder, more emetics, and bleeding, soothing potions, a plaster of pitch and pigeon dung on his feet, potions containing ten different substances, chiefly herbs, finally forty drops of extract of human skull, and the application of bezoar stones [animal gallstones then thought to be the crystallized tears of a deer bitten by a snake]; after which his majesty died (5).

Making a similar point in another framework, Miner wrote a classical whimsy called "Body Ritual Among the Nacirema" which appeared in an anthropological journal (6). He described a strange tribe which built into all their dwellings a pottery-walled shrine. Individuals went alone every morning and night into this shrine to perform various ablutions and body rituals. Evidence for the religious or cult nature of the shrine was found in a receptacle for fetishes and magic potions which occupied a prominent place in the shrine. When interrogated about the nature of these potions, the natives could not recall what most of the bottles were filled with, or when, where, or for what they were obtained. It would thus seem that they were retained in the receptacle for their general magical effect.

Nacirema is *American* spelled backwards; the shrine, the bathroom.

THE OPTION

The difficulties that lead patients into a physician's office for a placebo are assignable not to either the patient or the doctor but to the nature of the transaction between them. Perhaps a brief review of Samuel Butler's satire *Erewhon* can serve to introduce this point (7). When traveling in southern Italy in the nineteenth century, Butler noticed that the peasant subculture made no distinction between "would do something but medically cannot" and "medically can but won't." For example, the paraplegic with a transected spinal cord *cannot* walk though he would like to, whereas the malingerer with the same condition could walk but won't. This is a fundamental distinction in our society and one that has been incorporated into military regulations, school policy, and other official codes. In the peasant culture of Italy, Butler observed that a man who could not fulfill his assigned task for any reason, medical or moral, was left behind: he was regarded as dead wood. These observations may have led him to write his fictional account of an ideal society, Erewhon (an anagram of nowhere). Its mores were the converse of ours: medical illnesses were taboo and in fact criminal, while moral (that is, emotional) weaknesses were a common preoccupation and were treated by professionals called straighteners. The greeting "How are you?" could be politely answered by saying, "I've got a slight case of the socks," which was a highly formalized way of saying that one felt like shoplifting something of little value such as a pair of socks. This was meant to satirize our tendency to greet each other with a brief review of our medical complaints. In Erewhon, inevitable medical illnesses were hushed up by families since persons suffering them were sent off to jail. By portraying in the Erewhon society the opposite situation to that in our culture, Butler was pointing by indirection to the widespread use of medical illness in our society to cover problems with other people, groups of people, or institutions—what Butler called moral problems and what are now termed emotional problems.

Butler was sensitive to the social uses to which we put medical complaints and their real value in helping people cope with everyday problems and puzzles. Such observations can be carried one step further, literally into the medical clinic or office itself. It has been noted that people tend to make their problems into medical ones, regardless of whether they started out as such, because medical complaints are more socially acceptable, more "legitimate," more respectable, and more understandable to most of us than the vaguer problems of living that could be termed emotional or psychiatric. This transformation from generalized discomfort in living to medical complaint is in an extraordinarily large number of instances helped along by the unwitting or unheeding physician. When an impartial listener reports what frequently happens in the encounter of a new patient and doctor, it turns out that the former does not invariably or even frequently present complaints about a specific medical symptom or illness. For the most part, *patients offer an option* (8). They sit down, enact a variety of nonverbal expressions of distress and discomfort, and say something like this: "I'm having a great deal of trouble . . . and a backache." In most cases, medical doctors operate as a selective filter for medical complaints. When asked, they often openly state that they force the patient to discuss one and only one "medical" complaint per visit, not necessarily recognizing that by doing so they are excluding the problems in living that may have brought the patient to them in the first place. When confronted with this alternative, they generally can see their selective screening, but will indicate that they have no training or confidence in their ability to solve other kinds of problems in living even though the patient has given them the option. It has been reported that general practitioners extend this pessimism about intervening in nonmedical problems to the efforts of psychiatrists as well as themselves, and for this reason are reluctant to refer their patients to such specialists even if they identify their patients as having emotional problems (9, p. 30). In short, the medicalization of patients' complaints, with its attendant tremendous cost, is predicated on the failure of organized medicine to consider what a doctor does and how he does it. The widespread use of medical procedures such as a gall bladder X-ray series, for example, prescribed because of the doctor's inability and unwillingness to confront the patient's everyday unhappiness, is an irrelevant procedure at best and an appalling financial expense.

The presence of a sign of a disease such as a temperature does not mean that this sign is the determining factor which brings the patient to the doctor. Although patients do sometimes come to medical clinics because they have common colds, most people most of the time do not seek medical care for such an ailment; more critical if less readily stated reasons concern other medical or emotional fears or difficulties. To take a simple example, many people assume that doctors are going to reassure them automatically and not too convincingly if they speak of their worries and apprehensions; they have become immune to such reassurance. They postulate naively that if they go to a doctor and mention a minor complaint, the doctor is thus given the chance to notice other possible medical problems. If, however, the doctor does not comment on, say, the patient's hoarseness, then it must not be cancer as had been feared but merely a common cold after all. If the patient had asked about cancer directly he may have doubted the doctor's negative reply. Such reasoning is frequently characteristic of people requesting physical examinations. Here, then, is the other side of the coin; not only is it sometimes necessary to hide "emotional" complaints from the doctor by presenting them as an option, but medical problems as well are disguised.

There are three general outcomes to this kind of situation. First, almost anyone can produce some ailment—a little rash, a touch of diarrhea, a mild anxiety—that can be pressed into service by mutual agreement of doctor and patient to avoid a genuine discussion of life's problems. This is the "successful" outcome in the sense that the patient retains his dignity and his composure. But some unfortunate patients do not seem to be able to carry out this transaction adequately. They are either too vague—"I just feel funny"—or they produce a complaint which satisfies their family but is too unsophisticated for the doctor. When this happens, a subtle struggle may ensue between doctor and patient which not infrequently ends up in the patient being called a hysteric (8). In less common instances, the complaint that is ultimately formulated is clearly psychiatric, such as a phobia, and the patient is referred to a psychiatrist.

If there were someplace or someone to go to for help with ordinary unhappiness, the daily problems of living, there would probably be a sharp reduction in non-medically motivated visits to physicians and the distribution of pharmaceutical placebos. It is only recently that people have begun to accept the principle that "ordinary" unhappiness should in fact be tackled or treated. Freud assumed that resignation to the trials of life was the only solution. In many regions and eras, whole populations were resigned not only to the difficulties of daily life but to more radical illness processes such as malaria or schiztosomaisis (bladder parasite), as in Africa. Even today the average Egyptian peasant feels obliged to resign himself to these diseases, to learn to live with them rather than anticipate or demand their extirpation by social agencies or public facilities. It is perhaps a reflection of the relatively advanced level of Western science and medicine that we can today, in the context of community psychiatry, presume to intervene in the social and physical environments of those who feel oppressed by the ordinary problems they encounter. It has become evident that the apparently trivial and commonplace discomforts of daily living are not effectively handled by their translation into medical ideology, and it is necessary to provide some form of service where people can obtain relief, without disguise, for the troubles that prompt them to seek help.

In the absence of such facilities, people tend to convert their complaints into medical problems which they hope can be resolved by physicians. This illness process includes several progressive stages which have been analyzed by Balint (10) on the basis of seminars conducted with general practitioners. Following an initial period of vague perplexity, a lack of ease or dis-ease, the following developments are apt to ensue:

1. Intimate friends and relatives fail to help: "Particularly as a result of urbanization, a great number of people have lost their roots and connections, large families with their complicated and intimate interrelations tend to disappear, and the individual becomes more and more solitary, even lonely. If in trouble, he has hardly anyone to whom to go for advice, consolation, or perhaps only for an opportunity to unburden himself . . ." (10).

2. As a result of our cultural patterns, our familiarity with medical ideology, it is possible to become aware of bodily sensations that suggest a doctor may be helpful: "We know that in many people, perhaps in all of us, any mental or emotional stress or strain is either accompanied by, or tantamount to, various bodily sensations . . ." (10).

3. For lack of an alternative solution, one seeks out a physician: "In such troubled states . . . a possible and in fact frequently used outlet is to drop in to one's doctor and complain . . . it is here, in this initial, still 'unorganized' phase of an illness, that the doctor's skill is decisive . . ." (10).

4. At this point the patient offers the doctor the option, in one form or another: ". . . before they settle down to a definite 'organized' illness, he [the doctor] may observe that these patients, so to speak, *offer or propose various illness,* and they have to go on offering new illnesses until between the doctor and the patient an agreement can be reached, resulting in the acceptance by both of them of one of the illnesses as justified" (10).

If it is possible for the doctor to suggest other sources of the discomfort, or other places to go for help, illness does not follow in this sequence. For instance, when a health clinic was opened on the premises of a "little city hall" to which the public could take their social complaints, it was found that 60 percent of the medical patients were sent there instead of being treated for physical ailments. An earlier stage for intervention is at the beginning, the first step where the ordinary unhappiness can be talked about as such; if it is then alleviated, the final result is not necessarily a medical formulation. Finally, it must be noted that the type of agreement that occurs between doctor and patient depends upon the doctor's school of medicine; a chiropractor must negotiate a different agreement than an allopath.

The process that Balint delineates can go awry at any of the foregoing stages. In fact, in terms of solving the initial problem, the entire sequence can be seen as a failure. Agreement on a medical disease is a miscarriage in the face of more pressing problems of living, and so is agreement on a psychiatric disease. In both situations the original problem is further complicated rather than clarified. As Weinstein has noted:

> Recent studies of disability following industrial accidents illustrate an "accident process" in which social and emotional conflicts are resolved by substituting the "acceptable" disability of injury for the "unacceptable" disability of tension and depression. Aid to the Needy Disabled and other disability programs can become part of an analogous "illness process" in which medical impairment becomes the "acceptable" solution to a patient's longstanding conflicts in living. When disability programs serve this purpose, they vitiate efforts to reduce social and emotional tensions which really disable the patient. . . . Health professionals must learn how to help patients find less costly ways of coping with conflict than through the pseudo-solution of chronic disability (11).

This process can turn into an endless cycle, especially when patient and doctor fail to agree on a treatable medical complaint. Someone is vaguely distressed; because of lifelong contact with physicians, advertising, or other social influences he shapes his complaint in terms of a medical model. If this does not alleviate his distress, he eventually reaches a psychiatrist whose object, typically, is to transform his neurotic misery back into "ordinary unhappiness," as Freud expressed it. This transformation is sought using a model of individual psychology predicated on a medical model which cannot give adequate "meaning and form" to the problem, in Jung's terms. In the absence of a solution to his discomfort, the individual must seek another set of "healing fictions," which initiates a new cycle in the process.

THE HIDDEN AGENDA OF MEDICAL PRACTICE

The advanced surgical techniques and superb chemical treatments of contemporary medicine are about thirty years old. It is only since 1940 or so that medical treatment successfully copes with an enormous spectrum of disease. But if we examine a medical textbook published in 1900 (12), we can find for a disease such as rheumatoid arthritis the following remedies listed in the index:

baking cure	German cure
belladonna cure	home cure
camphor cure	Japanese cure
celery remedy	kerosene cure
crow-foot, for	lemon cure
electric cure	massage cure
wintergreen, for	water cure

None of these "cures" are in current use, nor could they possibly have been more than placebos in all those difficulties which used to be labeled as rheumatism. Evidently, medicine before 1940 survived on a small margin of successful intervention in disease processes. One may well ask what other function it did serve more effectively. Rather than bemoan the lack of efficacy of medicine of the previous centuries, we can consider the possibility that doctors were doing *something* successfully, something for which there was a need over and above the indisputable need to cure disease. In light of the foregoing discussion, one can say there was a hidden agenda—what Jung referred to as giving "meaning and form to the confusion" of the patient's mind.

Once one has broken through the curtain of silence about placebos, about the large proportion of unformulated problems in living that appear at the physician's doorstep, it becomes apparent that doctors have historically maintained the highest status in society despite the relative ineffectiveness of their medical techniques. Therefore they must have been doing something right. The role of placebos in sustaining the patient's faith is only one of the functions medicine seems to have fulfilled. The other major dimension, which has been veiled by a silence even more profound than that surrounding the placebo phenomenon, is that of medicine's role in social control and regulation. While this role becomes grossly obvious in its extreme and distorted application, as when the Soviet government disposes of obstreperous politicians and writers by sending them to mental hospitals, it is less apparent in the everyday process of medicalization of social problems which may be caused or exacerbated by slum housing, degrading welfare regulations, and so forth. In short, there seem to be *two* hidden agendas in the structure of medical practice: relief of cognitive dissonance or maintenance of faith in the possibility of resolving problems by use of placebos, and social control and regulation in the interest of maintaining the established political and social system.

Over the course of time in Western culture, disordered lives have routinely been seen as falling into one of five categories of deviance: sick, crazy, sinful, criminal, and resulting from social conditions. These are really the only major possibilities we have invented to categorize the various perplexities that befall us. The distribution has not always been equally divided between the five possibilities. In some centuries, for instance, religious explanations have predominated. To this day it is reported that 40 percent of people with emotional problems first seek help from the clergy (13). However, medicine now has a disproportionate number of referrals; the presumably scientific approach has displaced the religious in the orientation of most of us when we seek to account for deviant behavior. As we have noted, medicine as a system encourages the wide usage of medical and psychiatric channels and options, and the medicalization of problems in living.

In addition to the predominant patterns of thinking about behavioral disturbances that characterize a social group at a given time, there are a variety of subordinate contingencies that influence the classification of such behavior. Factors such as geographical location, skin color, social status, and educational level are recognized as sources of influence in the explanation of disturbed behavior. As is generally known, if one is sufficiently rich, the chances of being admitted to a neurological rather than psychiatric unit or being called eccentric rather than crazy are high. On the other hand, a lower-class Negro in a similar state of turmoil is apt to be seen, and see himself, as insane. Such labels and categories allow the machinery of society to process problems, and this in itself must be reassuring in some sense; everybody seems to know what is wrong and, hopefully, what to do about it. An analogous situation exists regarding the apparently straightforward issue of diagnosing crime. In this context, University of Michigan law professor Kamisar noted: "The white middle-class uses criminal codes as garbage cans. Whenever it has a problem it doesn't want to treat adequately, it draws up a criminal statute" (14). Prostitution, for example, can be seen as a complex psychiatric problem, a failing of the political or economic system, or simply a legal violation. Similarly, drug addiction can be seen as a disease, a moral failing, or a crime. More recently it has also been treated as a political problem by militant separatist ghetto groups who claim that they could abolish drug addiction if they could control their community and keep the drugs from entering their area.

As noted earlier, during the past several decades medicine has become, with the encouragement of its practitioners, a major solution to a wide array of problems in health and general welfare. However, some of these problems have gradually and recently become conceptualized in terms of community responsibility rather than within a traditional medical framework. In this newer view, a disordered life is regarded as the result of a failing of some function of society. Thus, a slum-dweller's lack of coping skills is seen as the outcome of his social context; the child once labeled schizophrenic is thought to have a disorganized family rather than a disorganized mind; a delinquent child is regarded no longer as essentially criminal, sinful, or crazy but as a mirror of the disorder and hopelessness of his environment; and a tuberculosis patient is regarded as suffering not only a failure of a lung but a failure of community hygiene.

It is unfortunate that formulations of problems in terms of community responsibility are inevitably related to political activity and activism. If physicians actually began to turn 60 percent of their practices away from their door, firmly believing that some element of community living was responsible and in need of revision to solve the problems patients were complaining about, political unrest would be greatly magnified. This is hardly the intention of any segment of the established order, much less a conservative group like physicians. Yet it becomes increasingly evident that adoption of the medical framework has a stabilizing political effect, in contrast to social diagnosis. It is also more socially acceptable to be ill than to be criminal, crazy, or morally deficient. The greater social stigma of the alternatives and the unavailability of agencies to handle and solve complaints formulated in their terms have further supported the widespread use of the medical option in diagnosing and treating a wide range of problems in living.

THE ECLIPSE OF THE MEDICAL OPTION

From the point of view of the social psychiatrist, the most striking change occurring today is the gradual eclipse of medicine's role as a catchall for problems. Whether or not this is viewed as a desirable trend, it is indisputably a dominant one. Despite the pressures and forces that have long upheld the medical model as the preferred format for the expression of so many kinds of problems of health and welfare, there is currently a distinct tendency to critically reconsider a medical construction of problems. Despite their lesser desirability and acceptability in the minds of many, the alternative categories of morality, the judicial process, and community organization are becoming increasingly important, both among intellectuals in their philosophical discussions, and among the poor and disadvantaged in their efforts to seek practical solutions to their everyday problems.

Within medicine itself, the increasing specialization that is coming about alters the nature of the physician-patient relationship and the role of medicine in solving problems. To a large extent, the specialist has become a highly skilled technician and researcher, while the general practitioner has become a highly skilled screener, broker, and advocate whose job includes representing his patients in their dealings with the complicated and relatively impersonal specialist systems. Although there exist varying degrees of generalist-specialist problems within one particular practice, the trend is toward a dichotomy. Accordingly, medicine at the specialist level becomes less ideological and by that token less "medical"; a very different kind of patient-doctor transaction ensues. As medicine becomes increasingly dichotomized, the field is transformed accordingly. The generalist becomes increasingly involved in community medicine and public health models in his thinking about medical problems and their solutions, and the specialist devotes more and more time to research. While the specialist studies problems of increasing specificity and narrowing of focus, the generalist and the community psychiatrists become concerned with the broader issues of the illness process, prevention, and environmental epidemiology. As the very nature of this chapter attests, the distinction between social psychiatry and the new breed of general practitioner immersed in community medicine declines in significance.

In psychiatry, this development is reflected theoretically in a move from inner space notions to outer space notions, from the study of mind to that of social behavior. In effect, social psychiatry thus appears to transfer its concerns from the medical (including psychiatric) category to that of community concerns. Family therapy provides an example of this change in point of view. One cannot consider family therapy a variety of medical-psychiatric treatment when it focuses on the social unit as the locus of the problem. At the same time it would be incorrect to see it as a really new approach. Rather, family therapy reflects a change in choice of *option* by therapist and family (doctor and patient) that had been previously available but seldom used— that is, a focus on social processes and communal involvement.

Thus in psychiatry as in medicine, there seems to be a current shift in conceptualization and construction of problems from a framework resting on the medical model of illness to a public health or social model. The latter entails political and community involvement which departs from the traditional function of medicine and physicians as stabilizers of the existing social order, and tends instead to lead to interest in social and political change and redistribution of power. Nevertheless, for pragmatic as well as philosophical reasons it is becoming increasingly apparent that the majority of problems suffered by the millions in our society are not amenable to cure from an exclusively medical point of view, that community involvement and political consciousness are inevitable components of their solutions.

ECOLOGICAL CONSCIOUSNESS

To define all problems in living as exclusively social or political would be as inaccurate as to define them all as medical; real problems tend to fall into more than one compartment. The task of classification is perhaps best approached by studying each of the categories as a more or less integrated system embracing ideology, professional agencies or workers, and practical outcomes. This would entail the observation of legal-judicial, medical, religious-moral, political, and psychiatric systems in terms of their separate functioning and also in terms of the multiple interactions between them.

Questions of interaction, influence, and balance between systems sharing a given environment or context represent focal issues of ecology. Their significance was first popularized by conservationists, whose early concern about the effect of one system on another stemmed from the fact that wildlife systems are among the most vulnerable and endangered in the organization of contemporary living. In the promotion of their interests, which generated limited public enthusiasm, they were able to arouse widespread attention by extending their argument to the general case, to all related systems. They demonstrated the thesis that the interdependence of various systems meant that when one was imperiled, the others were also. For example, many of the tidelands along the Eastern seaboard are disappearing as builders fill in these areas for industrial and housing uses. This has reduced the variety and number of wading birds, fish, and other fauna once endemic along the coast because this shallow water is a major nursery for young ocean fish. While the conservationists want to protect the remaining tidelands for bird-watching and other aesthetic purposes, they were able to demonstrate their importance for other systems, such as the fishing and shellfish industries, which are of greater practical and economic concern to the government. Ecological consciousness has thus become apparent among political and social groups concerned with the effects of physical and social systems on each other.

The same basic point of view is applicable to the illness process and the issue of pathogenesis. It is unlikely that one can see any situation clearly within a single framework, whether legal, medical, psychiatric, moral, or political. It is far more effective to examine the interactions between all of them. Crisis theory provides a means of theoretically coping with the large volume of data that inevitably is involved when multiples "fixes" are employed in the analysis of a given problem. Given a network of interconnected situations, any set of circumstances that disrupts what was previously going on can be viewed as a crisis: a time of opportunity and a time of danger. Any change, whether helpful or not, is then a crisis and tends to affect all other systems in the network under study. From the point of view of pathogenesis, the study of how a disease process begins, one must look for factors from any source in the complex network of systems within which one is operating in one's daily living.

Despite their theoretical attractiveness, ecological studies of problems in living are not easy to carry out, for a variety of reasons. First, most professionals are accustomed to approaching a given task within a specific and traditional framework taught to them in graduate school. When interdisciplinary conferences are held, these points of view and methods specific to only one profession are often suppressed or underplayed in the interest of interprofessional communication, leaving only those techniques and theories held in common. Thus instead of enriching the point of view held by each of the professional groups, interdisciplinary meetings tend to be geared to the lowest common denominator; the result is a lower level of functioning and communication than would occur within any of the participating professions, as Auerswald has shown (15). It is particularly unfortunate that assumptions about inner space and the use of an individual psychology are among the few concepts generally shared by interdisciplinary groups dealing with social problems, so that most explanations of behavior or illness attempted at all are formulated along these lines. This framework positively precludes adoption of an ecological framework and cannot show how people with problems weave their way between the various social systems, missing some or being waylaid by others. It is the very failure to negotiate with the various social systems that so often culminates in diagnosis of an illness, medical or psychiatric, and yet the processes by which this comes about cannot be observed except by adoption of the ecological model. To clarify this point further, it may be helpful to reconsider the subject of epigenetics.

THE SHAPE OF THE SOCIAL LANDSCAPE

The worst fate that could befall social psychiatry would be its identification as synonymous with political or social solutions to problems, whether those of the family or those of the state. As we have indicated, this would be merely shifting the emphasis from one institutional solution or system (psychiatry and medicine) to another (community responsibility). Social psychiatry proposes an overview, a superordinate point of view which examines the factors associated with all possible solutions. In order to present this point of view visually, it is possible to adapt Waddington's diagrams of embryology (16).

Let us imagine a landscape which is more or less undulating and tilted in such a fashion that a ball or marble would roll down it. Waddington refers to this as the "epigenetic landscape." The path followed by the ball as it follows one valley or another to the bottom corresponds to the developmental history of a problem. If one examines the diagram (Figure One), it can be noticed that trajectories of the ball starting from various points along the top edge find themselves converging on one or another of the valleys. Even if the ball is pushed slightly off its course, in a deep valley it will tend to compensate for such a disturbance and eventually reach the same end state that it would have normally. In general, end states are sharply distinct from each other.

In thinking in general about such landscapes, it is important to describe two factors: the tilt and the cross-section. The tilt at specific points will indicate the speed with which processes will occur. The cross-section will reveal, in the case of a deep valley, the degree of flexibility or the external force acting on the ball required to push it into a different valley.

There are three major types of landscapes corresponding to three major types of developments. The first landscape has deep

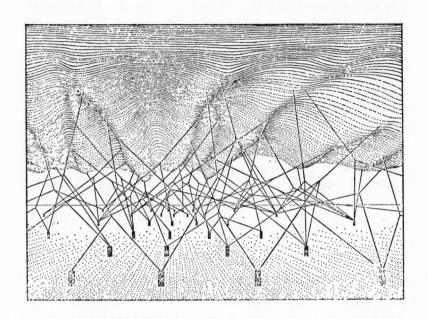

a

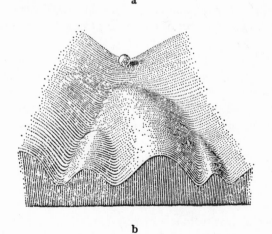

b

From *The Strategy of the Genes* by C. H. Waddington. George Allen & Unwin, Ltd., London, 1957, pp. 29, 36. Reprinted with the kind permission of the publisher.

valleys in it from the top to the bottom. This represents the type of career which is more or less determined from the start. A severe physical handicap is an example. In this case the definition and future development is more or less set and predictable. The second type of landscape starts off as rather undifferentiated and gradually takes on definite contours. This is essentially a gradient system starting with a tabula rasa which is more or less multipotential. The third type of landscape undergoes a change in the middle of the ball's downward travels, a landslide or some other change which grossly affects the cross-section or tilt. This represents a crisis.

In the situation we have been describing in medicine today the landscape is shaped in such a pattern that the valley that leads to a medical formulation is particularly deep and relatively easy to get into, whereas a religious formulation, for instance, is particularly difficult. The shift in the landscape being reported in this chapter is a deepening and increasing access to that valley that leads to a social or political formulation of a problem. The view that is particularly important to obtain is of the whole landscape, of all the valleys, even if one in particular is most frequently in use. In general one can say that however hard it may be to get into one of these valleys, it is even harder to get out. Becoming a welfare recipient, a psychiatric patient, an invalid, a religious fanatic, or a criminal all entail tendencies toward deep ruts.

The task of social psychiatry is to study the forces that shape the contours of the epigenetic landscape. If we imagine that the landscape is made of some material the underside of which is pulled by various ropes attached to it, thereby creating its shape, the task of social psychiatry is to understand how they work together (Figure One, b). It is here that the frontier lies.

SUMMARY

Many social institutions contribute to the control of socially unacceptable behavior. Medicine, its reputation and self-assessment notwithstanding, participates vigorously with all the rest in this endeavor by subtly shaping complaints and behavior which begin as either vague "dis-eases" or options in the direction of medical (i.e., physical) complaints. Psychiatric illness in this context merely represents a variant. A psychiatric diagnosis which is viewed with something less than respect by most doctors, such as "hysteria," may represent the culmination of a disagreement between doctor and patient or a discordance in the views of the doctor and the patient's social group as to what constitutes legitimate sick behavior. In other instances the doctor, the patient, and other significant people appear to be in agreement about controlling behavior that might otherwise be construed as a severe criticism of the social milieu; this is accomplished through a psychiatric construction of events in terms of which the patient is seen as failing to adjust to circumstances to which others have adjusted. The patient's mind is regarded as somehow deficient and in need of assistance or modification. The alternative proposition is that the individual's circumstances are unique, with a generalized epigenetic landscape; if adequately understood and evaluated, the so-called patient's behavior (or his position in the landscape) would be understandable without the need to resort to the metaphor of a failing mind.

CHAPTER NINE

Open Systems:
The Theory
of Treatment

> The philosopher has interpreted the world. The
> point, however, is to change it.
>
> KARL MARX

One of the basic objectives of social psychiatric treatment is the establishment of open and unimpeded
communication channels among members of natural groups. Initially this may seem unrelated to the major goal of psychoanalytic
treatment ("where id was, there shall ego be" [1, p. 112]), with its
stress on the achievement of impulse control and mastery by the
individual. However, the psychoanalytic tenet can be understood
as a specific instance of a broader category of events rather than
as a competitor that must be demolished to make room for social
psychiatric theory. It is the object of this chapter to compare both
the goals and general methods of the two therapeutic approaches
⁻–psychoanalysis and social psychiatry—within one area of the
general framework of communication theory. First the psychoanalytic vehicle of insight is compared to the social psychiatric use of
the concept of candor, and then the formal and substantive impli-

cations of blocked communications are considered. Mead's concept of significant communications is subsequently presented, together with an analysis of various categories of "awareness contexts" or the extent of impairment of communication channels. These categories include closed communication or secrets, suspected awarenesses, mutual pretense, and open communication (2). Finally, the function of self-knowledge in contrast to the acquisition of social competence is discussed, with a concluding section on the relevance of an educational model in psychotherapeutic undertakings.

Just as this summary of psychoanalytic treatment goals omits basic concepts such as transference, knowledge of which is vital to the psychoanalyst, the following discussion of the central issue of social psychiatric treatment will leave out many practical issues needed in a treatment situation. Such limitations are necessary precisely because the theoretical groundwork itself has not been laid and it is this subject to which the current chapter is addressed. The absence of such philosophical background creates certain dangers in current psychiatric practice. With the recent demand for social psychiatric services that both reach out to a broad cross-section of the population and are conducted within a brief time interval, there is a distinct peril of, as Bellak puts it, "a reversion to the preanalytic days of the common sense approach, the purely humane approach, which will involve the loss of the advantages of the valuable hypotheses that Freud applied" (3, p. 4). The mental health professional who rejects psychoanalysis in favor of a benevolent common sense runs the risk of functioning on the level of volunteer block worker. Such services are laudable and well meaning, but require no special skills or the extensive training and study that such professionals have already completed. It is the role of the professional to help evolve techniques and theory that can be applied to the practice of brief therapy, emergency therapy, community problems, and so forth. On the other hand, the therapist who attempts to apply orthodox psychoanalysis to such situations commits the opposite error of stifling an evolution from a psychoanalytic base to different method and theory more suited to the problems of natural groups.

In addition to developing and describing the central issue of the treatment of natural groups, that of the establishment and maintenance of open systems, this chapter will strive to relate psy-

choanalysis to social psychiatry somewhat differently, suggesting
that psychoanalytic explanations are subcategories of a more general situation not to be disproved by social psychiatry any more
than Einstein's relativity disproved Newton's mechanics. As Einstein himself suggested, "creating a new theory is not like destroy-
ing an old barn and erecting a skyscraper in its place. It is rather
like climbing a mountain, gaining new and wider views, discover-
ing unexpected connections. . . . But the point from which we
started out still exists . . . although it appears smaller and forms
a tiny part of our broad view" (4, p. 152).

INSIGHTS, CANDOR, AND CRUELTY

The notion of candor in social psychiatric theory replaces that
of insight in psychoanalytic theory as the major vehicle of therapeutic change. Adopting the more general framework of social
psychiatric theory, we can view the major problem areas in the
psychoanalytic theory of neurosis, such as the Oedipus complex
or castration anxiety, in terms of their formal characteristics as
well as their content. From this broader perspective, such issues
appear in their formal dimensions as failures in communication,
as family secrets with several variations. Some are really "open secrets" about which everybody is informed although the subject is
not discussed; others represent situations of "suspected awareness." Each of these categories represents a form of impaired communication, either blocked or distorted, and while the psychoanalyst would address himself to bringing about insight into their
content, the social psychiatrist is concerned with their form as representing failures in communication and their rectification
through achievement of candor rather than insight. In its time,
each approach has been termed cruel and ruthless on the part of
the therapist; the differences in social context and values between
Freud's Victorian Europe and contemporary America must be
considered in evaluating the relevance of such charges.

Today it is hard to imagine how Freud's ideas were received by
those who originally heard them. The Oedipus complex, for example, is now nicely packaged as one of the few secrets about
which we can all be singularly honest. By the same token, it is no

secret at all. Tortuous explanations of intellectual insight versus emotional insight have been invoked to account for the apparent indifference with which the Oedipus complex is greeted when it is "revealed" in its common form. Actually, the familiarity of most listeners with the content of such secret information seems a more probable reason for their failure to respond with Victorian emotion. Many subsidiary insights (penis envy, castration anxiety, vaginal dentata, and so forth) are essentially satellites of this one complex, and all have become acceptable or at least tolerable to the general public. The very fact that they are conceived as species-wide, generic problems is consoling for many. Yet when Freud first broached the topic of incest, it was considered by many a ruthlessly cruel thing to do. The Victorian climate was so unreceptive to most sexual discussion that in the case history of Katharina (5) published in 1900, Freud did not reveal for nearly twenty-five years that her seducer was the father and not a more distant relative. While Freud's emphasis in these situations was on the content, a sexual interest in the opposite-sex parent, it is also possible to focus on the form: family secrets. In this framework, the Oedipus complex can be regarded as a case where parents and children maintain secrets, where there is a failure of open communication. Before the reader is shocked by what he may construe as an endorsement of open sexual interest between parent and child, attention must be called to observations suggesting that children first learn about their attractiveness from the responses of their parents (6). It is not licentious for a father to communicate to his daughter an awareness that she is sexually attractive. In fact, it seems a daughter can only be protected by such knowledge, which encourages her to feel worthy of heterosocial and heterosexual encounters.

In the framework of social psychiatry, the nexus of pathology is seen as residing in the closed-off communication, not in the content, of the foregoing examples. What people must do to each other to so disrupt communication can be quite destructive, whether the secret is incest or something as mundane and trivial as bad breath. The disruption in communication can take several forms, entailing complete or partial silence. To refer again to the content of mutual sexual reactions within the family, fathers can withdraw from adolescent daughters who, having no idea that such behavior is related to their father's positive sexual response, begin to hate them for their sudden coldness. This condition would be one of "closed communication." A more damaging consequence can occur if there is partial leakage of the fathers' initial response, just enough to lead the daughter to have the "dirty thought" that there was something sexual involved. In this more complicated situation, there is not actually a secret but what could be called a "suspected awareness," which is even harder to cope with. Two points are noteworthy about such secrets: revealing them can be seen as cruel or painful, and they cover issues of behavior and not mental acts.

A third form that secrets can take is that of mutual pretense, and is illustrated by a story about the apparently trivial problem of bad breath. Bertrand Russell (7), in his autobiography, reported that his mistress of several years could not bring herself to tell him about his offensive breath and instead spoke of ending their relationship. As things turned out, Russell did consult a dentist during a trip to the United States, corrected the problem, and so saved his romance at the last moment. To understand this apparently simple anecdote, a more complicated view than his must be taken. It is exceedingly rare for someone to have chronic bad breath and not know it. In view of his subsequent actions, it seems apparent that Russell did know it, and therefore must have known that his mistress also knew it, although neither of them could deal directly with the matter. In fact she must have known that he knew of her awareness of the problem. It is in this curious state of affairs, which can occur with trivial as well as important matters, that communication channels can become blocked, that the disease processes discussed in the previous chapter can develop. In the current example, Russell probably thought that nothing could be done for his dental difficulties; this bit of ordinary unhappiness associated with despair about changing things led to a type of communication pattern that can be labeled mutual pretense.

While the issue of bad breath verges on humor, it cannot be denied that among the most profoundly brutal and exacting experiences we may undergo is the baring of our mutual pretenses. Revelation of such purposefully concealed information can have a disorganizing effect on the individual and his relationships even though its continued suppression entails discomfort and blocking of communication in a pathological sense. It has been argued that maintenance of such secrets is less disturbing to the status quo, and this is advocated by some even when the pathology involved is correctly identified. In this context the physician in Ibsen's *The Wild Duck* encourages the perpetuation of family or individual secrets, which he cynically refers to as the "vital lie":

Relling: Most of the world is sick, I'm afraid.
Gregers: And what's your prescription for Hjalmar?
Relling: My standard one. I try to keep the vital lie in him. . . . Deprive the average man of his vital lie, and you've robbed him of happiness as well (8, p. 202).

This all-too-common approach leaves a life surrounded by a thick wall of lethargy, "covered over with layers of dead skin, accumulations of habit, spontaneity buried under years of mechanical gestures. The living center is almost choked by debris and—what is worse—man has come to be content with living in the midst of this offal" (9, p. 11). Under such conditions, radical and typically painful intervention is required to bring about change, but in a therapeutic context this becomes the obligation of the therapist. In a parallel development, the theory of the Theatre of the Absurd expresses a similar idea—that the public must be unsettled, irritated, overpowered, and forced to react violently in order to react authentically. Writers like Cocteau, Gide, Adamov, Genet, and Beckett have tried to incorporate this premise in their work. To quote the playwright Antonin Artaud: "The word cruelty must be taken in a broad sense . . . cruelty signifies rigor, implacable intention and decision, irreversible and absolute determination" (9, p. 12). Although the American translation of Freud's insights were typically distorted to suggest that psychoanalysis was designed to provide happiness and pleasure, one finds the same approach in his writings:

I cannot recommend my colleagues emphatically enough to take as a model in psycho-analytic treatment the surgeon who puts aside all his own feelings, including that of human sympathy, and concentrates his mind on one single purpose, that of performing the operation as skillfully as possible. . . . The justification for this coldness in feeling in the analyst is that it is the condition which brings the greatest advantage to both persons involved. . . . An old surgeon once took for his motto the words: *Je le pansai, Dieu le guerit* [I bandage, nature cures]. The analyst should content himself with similar thoughts (10, p. 328).

In the strategy of effective therapy it is sometimes necessary to work on the assumption that the core of health in a family or other natural group is dangerously choked with the debris of mutual pretense and other forms of secrets. The initial objective then becomes the opening of communication channels and the abolition of secrets, regardless of either the content of the presenting problem or the apparent relevance of the secrets to these problems.

For a social psychiatrist, such revelations concern not inner matters of the mind but actual behavior. Two sources of error commonly appear to interfere with an understanding of what is meant by "actual behavior." First, individual psychology employs the concept of introjection to explain the influences of other people on the workings of the mind. Second, aspects of this "inner space" model are projected, so to speak, to account for the activities of social entities operating in the outer space of the environment.

Under the aegis of ego psychology, individual theory has incorporated many observations about the effect of social networks on behavior. For instance, when an inner structure such as the superego is postulated, one can say that the impact of influential people on the individual has been introjected, *taken into* the inner space of the model of mental structures. To account for the findings about reference groups in studies of social behavior, ego psychology has developed the notion of "superego nutriment" to include the idea that certain behaviors are needed for the maintenance of the inside structure. But the major emphasis of ego psychology is not on behavior; it is on the conceptual models that occupy the inner space of the individual. From the point of view of social psychiatry, this is an "error" that beclouds the meaning of behavior.

The second source of confusion lies in the application of inner space structures and concepts to groups inhabiting the outer space of the social world. Here, the inner organ is "projected" onto the outside world as an organism, a social organism. An example, cited in Chapter Seven, is putting a skin around an aspect of a network of people or things or places instead of leaving such a network as an unbounded and open system. A comparable error consists of applying the same processes used in inner space models to sociological or other psychological notions. For example, a mind *or* a family can be said to contain guilt. It seems to me that the imponderable substance of guilt is a liability of individual psychology and should be left there, since such a concept blocks inquiry about actual behavior. This error of allowing the imponderable affects to spill over into other areas is also apparent in certain sociological thinking. For instance, a gang may be seen as having within it something labeled social pressure, which is seen as the explanation for obedience to gang rules.

To clarify the kind of error that such thinking entails, the example of gang influence can be pursued. Instead of the idea of an imponderable affect to explain behavior, actual studies of events can be carried out. It can then be observed that if a boy does not follow gang rules, wants to leave the gang, or refuses to join it, the other members are apt to enact disciplinary measures such as framing him for a crime or deliberately getting him into trouble. Once he has a police record, possibilities of leaving the gang are reduced. Milder gang influence can be expressed in the form of practical jokes. Such coercion or threat of violence is hardly as mysterious as "social pressure" sounds, and deserves to be considered directly. Imponderables merely make the world around us less amenable to observation, understanding, and active intervention. In short, the introjection of observations about social influences to inner space formulations and the projection of structures and concepts of individual psychology together serve to obscure the actual behavior that takes place among the people one is interested in understanding.

To summarize the major points noted above: the notion of insight in psychoanalytic theory is considered to be replaced by that of candor in social psychiatric theory. By candor is meant honesty or accurate observation about what men do or are disposed to do to each other. Adoption of this strategy may entail the opening by the social psychiatrist of a Pandora's box of all the inhuman things that humans do to each other, but it is believed to facilitate behavioral change and eventual reestablishment of open and healthy patterns of communication.

SIGNIFICANT COMMUNICATIONS AND
AWARENESS CONTEXTS

What any two people know about each other and what each knows the other knows about him is a hard issue to put into words. In philosophical terms it has been expressed as "the knowledge of other intelligences," the opposite of solipsism, and Mead has used the term "significant communications." In his introduction to the subject he wrote: "Sometimes we find that we can best think out an argument by supposing that we are talking to somebody who takes one particular side. . . . In that way in the night hours we are apt to go through distressing conversations we have to carry out the next day. That is the process of thought. *It is taking the attitude of others,* talking to other people, and then replying in their language. That is what constitutes thinking" (11, p. 33; italics mine). In more contemporary terminology, *feedback* might be used to describe what Mead had in mind. For him the adjustment of the second person or listener in response to the communicative gesture of the first person or speaker gives the latter's gesture the meaning it has. Meaning may thus be seen as a relationship between certain phases of social actions; it is not a mental addition to an act but itself constitutes a feedback loop of communicative behavior.

In contrast to human communication where such feedback exists, animal communication provides a simpler form: when an animal brings about a meaning for another animal, he is not simultaneously bringing about the same meaning for himself. For the animal, the listener's response is not necessarily relevant or of significance to the speaker or the sender of the message. Such communication occurs without awareness of the real effect on the receiving animal. Such simple communication can be found in insect communities, in which signals are sent regardless of the need, as in situations without receivers or in which the message has been delivered many times before. Thus a bee may signal the direction of honey to an empty hive.

The more complex communication condition exists when a gesture may lead to an adjustment in the receiver and also in the sender himself. In this situation one might say that the sender becomes a receiver of his own message. For example, if a gesture we make evokes a certain response in another person or a network of people and we are aware of that response (which is a response to us), the effect of the attitude that we produce in the network comes back to ourselves in a feedback loop. We become aware of ourselves from the standpoint of others. In this sense it seems that first we know others, and then we are able to put ourselves in their place. By taking the position of the other toward ourselves, we become an observer of ourselves—what Mead called a "me" to an "I." We enter our own experience as an individual not directly but only insofar as we first become an observer to ourselves. A gesture becomes *significant* when we think about the response of *significant* others to it. Mead referred to this complicated gesture as a "significant gesture." The point of view is similar to that of Marx: "The general result at which I arrived and which, once won, served as a guiding thread for my studies, can be briefly formulated as follows: in the social production of their life, men enter into definite relations that are indispensable and independent of their will. . . . [this] conditions the social, political, and intellectual life process in general. It is not the consciousness of men that determines their social being, but, on the contrary, their social being that determines their consciousness" (12, p. 362–64). In other words, for both Mead and Marx consciousness can be totally equated with self-consciousness—with the awareness of the effect of our behavior on significant others.

This orientation provides us with a theoretical framework in which to consider awareness contexts. Neither Mead nor Marx spent much time considering how such sophisticated communication develops. They simply assumed that it would develop in the course of each person's maturation. To some extent such an assumption is naive in that it overlooks miscarriages of the developmental process: if we assume that communication patterns develop, we must also allow for the possibility that they develop badly, or wrongly, and it is here that the question of social pathology manifests itself.

Sullivan was probably the first psychiatrist to consider such miscarriages, or warps, as he called them, of the normal development of communication skills in relation to the subsequent emergence of disturbed behavior. He was particularly interested in the general need to experience situations of mutual intimacy and candor permitting the cross-validation of personal worth; that is, where another's admiration and respect is openly communicated and serves to enhance one's feelings of self-esteem. He observed that this experience is not available to everyone, and certainly does not prevail most of the time; people hide and dissemble as much as they reveal about themselves and their feelings towards others. Sullivan thought he found in early adolescence a fairly typical developmental phase where this kind of ideal communication pattern does exist between "chums," when one has a very special tie with a friend of the same sex in which conscious intimacy can take place. Sullivan defined intimacy in terms of Mead's idea of consciousness: intimacy is said to occur when another reflects yourself to you as he actually experiences you, and vice versa, with the eventual outcome of mutual acceptance. In his clinical studies, Sullivan noted that this experience of intimacy during the formative years was virtually a prerequisite to healthy adjustment in later life, and its absence constituted a poor prognostic sign among the "schizophrenics" he treated.

Mead's editor, Strauss, has subsequently studied clinical variations of what Mead would term "significance." As noted, a gesture becomes significant when we are aware of the responses of other people to it. There are many gradations possible. Working with Glaser, Strass (2) has defined several "awareness contexts" based on a study of communication patterns between hospital staff members and dying patients and of conditions of hospital organization that influence such transactions. Awareness contexts are basically defined in terms of what each interacting person knows of the patient's status (proximity to death) as well as the awareness each has of the other's awareness of the patient's status —i.e., who knows what and what each knows about what others know. Glaser and Strass delineate four major categories or contexts: closed, suspected, mutual pretense, and open. Since these categories are related to the preceding discussion of insight vs. candor in various psychotherapeutic treatment strategies, each will be considered in some detail.

Closed awareness contexts are secrets. A secret, to be a secret, must make absolutely no difference, which is more unlikely than is usually thought. Freud once remarked: "He that has eyes to see and ears to hear may convince himself that no mortal can keep a secret. If his lips are silent, he chatters with his finger-tips; betrayal oozes out of him at every pore" (13, p. 94). The likelihood of observing discrepancies between verbal and nonverbal behavior can be demonstrated by turning off the sound of a television drama; without the dialogue, the behavior usually is unconvincing. Most actors err in the direction of making too many gestures. Scheflen (14) has said that the location of the "unconscious" lies in the disparity between verbal and postural-kinesic aspects of communication. In short, most of us are apt to reveal attitudes, opinions, and information even if we want to keep them secret and think we are doing so. In contrast, it is relatively easy for natural groups to keep secrets within their own networks. Information tends to stop at certain interfaces, not because of special efforts or skills on the part of network members but because beyond a given point there are no others who care about the particular secret. It makes no difference to someone to hear confidential information about a total stranger, and no difference to the stranger. Therefore, although one could very easily be told such a secret (because it makes no difference), the chances are that it will not be passed on. It is probably the irrelevance of secrets to total strangers that makes patients willing to have psychotherapy sessions taped or filed for future observation by unknown colleagues of their therapists.

Suspected awareness contexts have been previously mentioned in relation to the girl who has the "dirty thought" that her father may be sexually aroused by her. In such situations the uncertainty itself can be quite destructive since there is always the possibility that one may be wrong and that such suspicion stems from one's own mental illness or perversion, or something equally frightening. Unless the girl in this situation is very much aware that fallibility is normal and requires no explanation or justification, she may have too much at stake, may be too fearful of the consequences, to check out her suspicions in order to verify or disprove them.

In psychoanalytic theory it is held that an affect attached to an unconscious idea operates more strongly, and since it cannot be inhibited, is potentially more injurious than an affect attached to a conscious idea (15, p. 61). It has already been suggested that suspected awareness contexts operate in similar fashion. Because the thought cannot be expressed and validated or rejected, it can assume all sorts of distorted forms and a seriousness that it might not have if it were in the open. It appears that the psychoanalytic concept is a special case within the general area of awareness contexts. It is not that social psychiatry must replace "repression" as an explanation but that it can be seen within a wider field of concern.

Mutual pretense is a more complicated set of circumstances than the psychoanalyst takes into account with the concept of repression or the social psychiatrist with that of suspected awareness. Perhaps the concept of mutual pretense could be encompassed within a liberal, neo-Freudian theory of transference and countertransference. It cannot be a function of a single individual but must involve two or more. For example, a father can know that his daughter was pregnant before her marriage, but when he tells the story to a therapist in the presence of his family, the fact can slip his mind and not be mentioned by anyone else. If such mutual pretenses characterize the general state of the family, each member must act a part that is not genuine. This requires a talent for acting or, more probably, the invention of many excuses such as medical illness. Furthermore, whole areas of discourse and recollection must be avoided. In fact the situation is such that the prevailing transactions are going on with make-believe characters each nursing a "vital lie." Recognition of the pregnancy would be less damaging than an effect of this nature. In another clinical example, a father had two wives and was legally a bigamist. His son was never told and did not speak of it, but he knew about the matter. In a third family, the nominal or index patient was a depressed wife; here, the mutual pretense disguised the husband's struggle with homosexual impulses. The therapists were not told about this openly, although every member of the extended family had at one time or another been confidentially told that this husband had approached other members. Many family members worried that the husband might also approach his own young sons. Another situation of mutual pretense often surrounds terminal illness. If someone is dying and knows it and those around him know it too, the ensuing social transaction, if all pretend ignorance, becomes disastrous. In interviews of children in terminal stages of leukemia, some refer to the experience of living in such a mutual-pretense system as being dead already. In each instance, a great deal of strange behavior must occur to avoid open communication. In such cases psychotherapy begins with "spilling the beans." (In Chapter Two the technique of obtaining permission or a "release" to proceed along such lines was briefly described.)

PESSIMISM OR OPTIMISM

Mutual pretense is not the exclusive province of patients. The psychotherapeutic profession, including social psychiatry, is forever claiming skills it does not have and delineating achievements that are not presently realistic in terms of the current knowledge and facilities available. At the same time such pretenses are comforting, and it is hard to demand that patients do something the profession itself finds difficult to do. It seems abundantly clear that there are very few indisputable data available about the treatment of disordered lives, and it would seem that professional pretense about such matters will only be reflected in equivalent deceptions by patients. Would a confession of limitation and inability heal pain? Would it advance the frontiers of a just society? Let us not claim too much for such candor, but suggest that it may promote higher standards of ethics and thoughtfulness.

An essential difference between psychoanalytic and social psychiatric points of view concerns this issue of pessimism and optimism. Freud argued that the world shapes man through assaults on his inner life. In Freudian theory, the high payoff is a lonely wresting of individual gratification from a hostile world. Dewey and other social theorists argued, in contrast, that man makes himself. As Rieff has said, "Dewey and Freud meet back-to-back" (15, p. 32). Dewey accused Freud of reducing social results to psychic causes. For Freud there is no point in trying to change the world, including the behavior of individuals toward each other, because man's essential dilemmas are inborn and inevitable. On the other hand, if Marx's metaphor has validity and we are confusing what man makes with what makes man, if these dilemmas are actually made by men and can be changed by men, then there is room for limited optimism. It is noteworthy that the more pessimistic psychoanalytic view, at least in its American version, is associated with claims that emphasize the enormous pow-

ers of psychiatric treatment, while the more optimistic view is as
sociated with a more modest assessment.

KNOWING HOW AND KNOWING THAT

The individual psychology model envisions psychotherapy as a
two-stage operation: first the patient must mentally grasp a certain insight, and then he must on his own change his behavior accordingly via some vague neurological connection between mind
and body. While the mind-body problem itself should tend to dis-
courage such a formulation, Ryle (16) has criticized the notion
that knowing *that* preceeds knowing *how*, that insight precedes
competence. If every act must be preceded by the prior awareness
of rules, propositions, or insights, then we must ask how it is possible to achieve this task of prior awareness (insight-ing). The
only answer consistent with individual theory is that we must
contemplate other rules, propositions, and insights about rules,
propositions, and insights. Since the very same question may be
asked about these second-order rules, propositions, and insights,
we must have a third, fourth, and so forth ad infinitum. It
would be impossible ever to do an intelligent thing. Since this infinite regress is obviously absurd, another answer must be sought.

Ryle proposed that social competence be seen as an alternative
model to insight: "When a person is described by one or other of
the intelligence-epithets such as 'shrewd' or 'silly' . . . the description imputes to him not the knowledge, or ignorance, of this
or that truth, but the ability, or inability, to do certain
things. . . . In ordinary life . . . we are much more concerned
with people's competences than with their cognitive repertoires"
(16, pp. 27–28). Ryle is here observing that when we say someone
does something intelligently, we mean that he does it well—that
the act is competent, not that it has intelligent antecedents.

Ryle's point of view shows itself in social psychiatric theory as a
concern for behavioral change rather than theoretical change or
the achievement of insights. In the example of a conflict between
two people, the question is what tasks are necessary to resolve
their dispute, not what special insights about it must be contem-
plated. One might suggest such a mundane effort as sitting next

to each other and thinking of three positive things about the other person. Any interpretation used in obtaining this result—conflict resolution—is really a power move. Thus if I am told that I am fighting with someone because I'm really angry with my father because of his exclusive sexual rights to my mother, I am being pressured to end the fight. If I do so, it will be not because of the insight so revealed but as the result of pressure brought upon me to perform whatever tasks will end the fight. The change that transpires does not actually have two stages: first the contemplation of certain truths, and then the performance of certain behavior. The two are part of the same act. It is therefore the special competence of the social psychiatrist to examine the complex behavior that occurs within natural groups and then prescribe those tasks that must take place for the desired change to come about.

References

Chapter One. Introduction: The New Science

1. Bell, N. W., and Spiegal, J. P.: Social Psychiatry. *Arch. Gen. Psychiat.* 14:337–345, 1966.

2. G. A. P. Committee on Medical Education: *The Pre-clinical Teaching of Psychiatry.* Report No. 54, New York, October 1962.

3. Hobbs, N.: Mental Health's Third Revolution. *Amer. J. Orthopsychiat.* 34:822–833, 1964.

4. Whittington, H. G.: The Third Psychiatric Revolution—Really? *Comm. Ment. Health J.* 1:73–80, 1965.

5. Schulberg, H. C., and Baker, F.: Varied Attitudes to Community Mental Health. *Arch. Gen. Psychiat.* 17:658–663, 1967.

6. Dunham, W.: Community Psychiatry: The Newest Therapeutic Bandwagon. *Arch. Gen. Psychiat.* 12:303–313, 1965.

7. Strauss, A., Bucher, R., Ehrlich, D., Schatzman, L., and Sabshin, M.: *Psychiatric Ideologies and Institutions.* New York: Free Press, 1964.

8. Srole, L. Social Psychiatry: A Case of the Babel Syndrome. Read before the American Psychopathological Association, New York, February, 1967.

9. Rapaport, D.: The Structure of Psychoanalytic Theory: A Systematizing Attempt. *Psychol. Issues,* No. 6, 1960. Also in S. Koch, ed.: *Psychology: A Study of a Science,* vol. 3. New York: McGraw-Hill, 1959, pp. 55–183.

10. Kazin, A.: *Contemporaries.* Boston: Little, Brown, 1962.

11. Joint Commission on Mental Illness and Health (1960): *Action for Mental Health.* New York: Sciences Editions, 1961.

12. Bergin, T. G., and Fisch, M. H., trans.: *The New Science of Giambattista Vico.* New York: Anchor Books, 1961.

13. Harris, F. R.: National Social Science Foundation: A Proposed Congressional Mandate for the Social Sciences. *Amer. Psychol.* 22:904–910, 1967.

14. Davis, V.: Testimony before the Subcommittee on Government Research, Committee on Government Operations, United States Senate, 90th Congress, 1st Session, June 21, 1967.

15. McLuhan, M.: *Understanding Media: The Extensions of Man.* New York: McGraw-Hill, Paperbacks, 1966.

16. Lawson, G. L., ed.: *Orthopsychiatry, 1923–1948, Retrospect and Prospect.* New York: American Orthopsychiatric Association, 1948.

17. Jenkins, R., and Cole, J., eds.: *Diagnostic Classification in Child Psychiatry.* New York: American Psychiatric Association, 1964.

18. Rieff, P.: *Freud, the Mind of the Moralist.* New York: Viking, 1959.

19. Smolen, E. M., and Rosner, S.: Observations on the Use of a Single Therapist in a Child Guidance Clinic. *J. Amer. Acad. Child Psychiat.* 2:345–356, 1963.

20. Brody, E. B.: Continuing Problems in the Relationship between Training in Psychiatry and Psychoanalysis in the U.S.A. *J. Nerv. Ment. Dis.* 136:58–67, 1963.

21. Mailer, N.: *New York Times,* August 4, 1968, p. 58.

22. Southard, E. E., and Jarrett, M. C.: *The Kingdom of Evils.* New York: Macmillan, 1922.

23. Bockoven, J. S.: *Moral Treatment in American Psychiatry.* New York: Springer, 1963.

24. Goldhamer, H., and Marshall, A. W.: *Psychosis and Civilization: Two Studies in the Frequency of Mental Disease.* Glencoe, Ill.: The Free Press, 1949.

25. Sarason, S. B., Levin, M., Goldenberg, I., and Cherlin, D. L.: *Psychology in Community Settings.* New York: Wiley, 1966.

26. Bell, D.: The Year 2000—The Trajectory of an Idea. *Daedalus* 96:639–651, 1967.

27. Kopkind, A.: The Future-Planners. *Amer. Psychol.* 22:1036–1041, 1967.

28. Laswell, H.: What Psychiatrists and Political Scientists Can Learn From One Another. *Psychiatry* 1:33–40, 1938.

29. Pirie, N.W.: Concepts Out of Context: The Pied Pipers of Science. *Brit. J. Phil. Sci.* 2:269–280, 1952.

30. Snell, B.: *The Discovery of the Mind.* New York: Harper Torchbooks, 1960.

31. Jones, E.: *The Life and Work of Sigmund Freud,* vol. 2. New York: Basic Books, 1955.

32. Rapaport, D., and Gill, M.: The Points of View and Assumptions of Metapsychology. *Int. J. Psychoanal.* 60:153–162, 1959.

33. Gill, M., and Brenman, M.: *Hypnosis and Related States.* New York: International Universities Press, 1959, pp. 202–218.

Chapter Two. Inner and Outer Space: Dynamics

1. Whorf, B. L.: *Language, Thought and Reality.* Cambridge, Mass.: M.I.T. Press, 1956.

2. Snell, B.: *The Discovery of the Mind.* New York: Harper Torchbooks, 1960.

3. Onians, R. B.: *The Origins of European Thought about the Body, the Mind, the Soul, the World, Time and Fate.* Cambridge, England: Cambridge University Press, 1951.

4. Kitto, H. D. F.: *The Greeks.* Baltimore: Penguin Books, 1951.

5. Sarbin, T.: Anxiety: Reification of a Metaphor. *Arch. Gen. Psychiat.* 10:630–638, 1964.

6. Rieff, P. *The Triumph of the Therapeutic.* New York: Harper & Row, 1966.

7. Vygotsky, L. S.: *Thought and Language.* New York: John Wiley and M.I.T. Press, 1962.

8. Mills, C. W.: *Sociology and Pragmatism.* New York: Galaxy Books, 1966.

9. Strauss, A., ed.: *The Social Psychology of George Herbert Mead.* Chicago: University of Chicago Press, 1956.

10. Chappell, V. C.: *The Philosophy of Mind.* Englewood Cliffs: Prentice Hall, 1962.

11. Benjamin, B. S.: Remembering. In D. F. Gustafson, ed., *Essays in Philosophical Psychology.* New York: Doubleday, 1964, pp. 171–194.

12. Freud, S.: The Future Prospects of Psychoanalytic Therapy. In *The Standard Edition of the Complete Psychological Works of Sigmund*

Freud. London: Hogarth Press and the Institute of Psycho-Analysis, 1957, Vol. 11, 141–142.

13. Hart, H.L.A.: The Ascription of Responsibility and Rights. In A. G. N. Flew, ed., *Logic and Language* (First Series). Oxford: Basil Blackwell, 1951, pp. 145–166.

Chapter Three. Heat, Electricity, and Love: Dynamics

1. Singer, C.: *A Short History of Scientific Ideas to 1900.* London: Oxford University Press, 1959.

2. Maxwell, J. C.: Preface, *Matter and Motion.* New York: Dover, n.d.

3. Freud, S.: The Defence Neuropsychoses, *Collected Papers,* Vol. 1. London: Hogarth Press, 1953.

4. Freud, S.: *Group Psychology and the Analysis of the Ego.* New York: Liveright, 1951.

5. Freud, S.: *The Problem of Anxiety.* New York: Norton, 1936.

6. Barber, T. X.: Toward a Theory of Pain Relief: Relief of Chronic Pain by Prefrontal Leucotomy, Opiates, Placebo and Hypnosis. *Psychol. Bull.* 6:430–460, 1959.

7. Bedford, E.: Emotions, in V. C. Chappell, ed., *The Philosophy of Mind.* Englewood Cliffs: Prentice-Hall, 1962.

8. Ryle, G.: *The Concept of Mind.* New York: Barnes and Noble, 1949.

9. Sullivan, H. S.: *The Interpersonal Theory of Psychiatry.* New York: Norton, 1953.

10. Bateson, G., Jackson, D., Haley, J., and Weakland, J.: Toward a Theory of Schizophrenia. *Behav. Sci.* 1:251–264, 1959.

11. Dewey, J. and Bentley, A. F.: *Knowing and the Known.* Boston: Beacon Press, 1957.

12. Strauss, A., ed.: *The Social Psychology of George Herbert Mead.* Chicago: University of Chicago Press, 1956.

13. Hart, H. L. A.: The Ascription of Responsibility and Rights. In A. G. N. Flew, ed. *Logic and Language* (First Series). Oxford, Basil Blackwell, 1951, pp. 145–166.

14. Austin, J. L.: Other Minds. In A. G. N. Flew, ed., *Logic and Language* (Second Series). Oxford: Basil Blackwell, 1953.

15. Leifer, R.: The Psychiatrist and Tests of Criminal Responsibility.

Amer. Psychol. 19:825–830, 1964.

16. Szasz, T.: *The Myth of Mental Illness.* New York: Hoeber, 1961.

17. Goffman, E.: The Moral Career of the Mental Patient. *Psychiatry* 22:123–142, 1959.

18. Haley, J.: The Art of Being Schizophrenic. *Voices* 1:133–147, 1965.

19. Block, D. A., and Rosenthal, R. A.: Psycho-Social Replication. Paper read at First International Congress of Social Psychiatry, London, August 1964.

20. Lennard, H. L., Beaulieu, M. R., and Embrey, N. G.: Interaction in Families with a Schizophrenic Child. *Arch. Gen. Psychiat.* 12:166–183, 1965.

21. Rabkin, R.: Conversion Hysteria as Social Maladaptation. *Psychiatry* 27:349–363, 1964.

22. Warkartin, J.: Editorial. *Voices* 1:4, 1965.

Chapter Four. Topography: Is the Unconscious Necessary?

1. Descartes, R. In N. K. Smith, trans.: *Descartes' Philosophical Writings.* London: MacMillan, 1962.

2. Plato. In B. Jowett, trans.: *The Dialogues of Plato.* London: Oxford University Press, 1931.

3. May, R.: The Psychoanalyst's Motivation to Help. Panel discussion, *Contemp. Psychoanal.* 1:38–44, 1964.

4. Peirce, C. S. In C. Hartshorne and P. Weiss, eds.: *The Collected Papers of Charles Saunders Peirce,* vol. 5. Cambridge, Mass.: Harvard University Press, 1931–1935.

5. Gallie, W. B.: *Peirce and Pragmatism.* Marmondsworth, Middlesex: Penguin Books, 1952, pp. 59–83.

6. Holt, R. R.: Freud's Cognitive Style. *Amer. Imago* 22:163–179, 1965.

7. Freud, S.: *A General Introduction to Psychoanalysis.* New York: Permabooks, 1953.

8. Freud, S. Quoted in E. Jones, *The Life and Work of Sigmund Freud,* vol. 2. New York: Basic Books, 1955.

9. Foulkes, D.: Theories of Dream Formation and Recent Studies of Sleep Consciousness. *Psychol. Bull.* 62:236–247, 1964.

10. Jones, R.: *Ego Synthesis in Dreams.* Cambridge, Mass.: Schenk-

man, 1962.

11. Wiener, P. P., ed.: *Values in a Universe of Chance: Selected Writings of Charles S. Peirce.* New York: Doubleday Anchor, 1958, pp. 101, 351, 398, 426.

12. Antrobus, J. S., Antrobus, J. S. and Fisher, C.; Discrimination of Dreaming and Nondreaming Sleep. *Arch. Gen. Psychiat.* 12:395–401, 1965.

13. Hawthorne, N.: *The House of Seven Gables.* New York: New American Library, 1961.

14. Popper, K. R.: On the Source of Knowledge and Ignorance. *Encounter* 19:42–57, 1962.

15. Neitzsche, F. Quoted in L. L. Whyte: *The Unconscious Before Freud.* New York: Basic Books, 1960.

16. Dewey, J. *The School and Society.* Chicago: University of Chicago Press, 1909.

17. Kazin, A.: *Contemporaries.* Boston: Little, Brown, 1962.

18. Sullivan, H. S.: *Schizophrenia as a Human Process.* New York: Norton, 1962.

19. Sanford, R. N.: The Development of the Healthy Personality in the Society of Today. In *Modern Health Concepts and their Application in Public Health Education,* No. 8, Berkeley, Calif.: State Department of Public Health, 1959.

20. Vygotsky, L. S.: *Thought and Language.* New York: John Wiley and M.I.T. Press, 1962.

21. Henry, J.: *Culture Against Man.* New York: Vintage Books, 1963.

Chapter Five. The Shape of Time: Epigenetics

1. Moor, A. A. Quoted in *The New York Times,* March 18, 1965.

2. Bridgeman, P.: *The Way Things Are.* Cambridge, Mass.: Harvard University Press, 1959.

3. Whorf, B. L.: *Language, Thought and Reality.* Cambridge, Mass.: M. I. T. Press, 1956.

4. Onians, R. B.: *The Origins of European Thought about the Body, the Mind, the Soul, the World, Time and Fate.* Cambridge, England: University of Cambridge Press, 1951.

5. Homer: *Iliad.* Trans. W. H. Rouse. New York: Mentor, 1950.

6. Draper, T.: Vietnam: How Not to Negotiate. *New York Review*

of *Books* 8:17–29, May 4, 1967.

7. Watts, A.: *The Way of Zen.* New York: Pantheon, 1957.

8. Aries, P.: *Centuries of Childhood: A Social History of Family Life.* New York: Knopf, 1962.

9. Gioscia, V.: On Social Time II. In H. Osmond, H. Jaker and F. Cheek, eds., *Man's Place in Time.* New York: Doubleday, 1969.

10. Mailer, N.: The White Negro. In *Advertisements for Myself,* New York: Putnam, 1959.

11. Camus, A.: *The Stranger.* Trans. S. Gilbert. New York: Knopf, 1946.

12. Jones, R. M.: *Ego Synthesis in Dreams.* Cambridge, Mass.: Schenkman, 1962.

13. Erikson, E.: *Childhood and Society.* New York: Norton, 1950.

14. Beach, F. A.: Characteristics of Masculine "Sex Drive." In M. R. Jones, ed., *Nebraska Symposium on Motivation 1956.* Lincoln: University of Nebraska Press, 1956, pp. 1–32.

15. McLuhan, M.: *Understanding Media: The Extensions of Man.* New York: McGraw-Hill, 1965.

16. de Laguna, F.: *The Study of a Tlingit Community: A Problem in the Relationship between Archeological, Ethnological and Historical Methods.* Washington D.C.: U.S. Government Printing Office, 1960.

17. Gill, M. M., and Rapaport, D., The Points of View and Assumptions of Metapsychology. In M. M. Gill, ed., *The Collected Papers of David Rapaport.* New York: Basic Books, 1967, pp. 795–811.

18. Dennis, N.: *Cards of Identity.* New York: Vanguard, 1955.

19. Strauss, A. ed.: *The Social Psychology of George Herbert Mead.* Chicago, University of Chicago Press, 1956.

20. Goffman, E.: *Asylums.* New York: Anchor, 1961.

Chapter Six. Energy: Economics

1. Freud, S.: Project for a Scientific Psychology. In *The Origins of Psychoanalysis.* New York: Basic Books, 1954.

2. du Bois-Reymond, E. Quoted in S. Bernfeld, Freud's Earliest Theories and the School of Helmholtz. *Psychoanal. Quart.* 13:341–362, 1944.

3. Holt, R. R.: Beyond Vitalism and Mechanism: Freud's Concept of Psychic Energy. *Science and Psychoanalysis,* vol. II. New York: Grune

and Stratton, 1967, pp. 1–41.

4. Ostow, M. Quoted in A. H. Modell, The Concept of Psychic Energy, *J. Amer. Psychoanal. Ass.* 11:605–618, 1963.

5. Singer, C.: *A Short History of Scientific Ideas to 1900.* London: Oxford University Press, 1959.

6. Dewey, J., and Bentley, A. F.: *Knowing and the Known.* Boston: Beacon Press, 1949.

7. Ginsberg, A.: A Reconstructive Analysis of the Concept "Instinct." *J. Psychol.* 33:235–277, 1952.

8. Schneirla, T. C.: Behavioral Development and Comparative Psychology. *Quart. Rev. of Biol.* 41:283–302, 1966.

9. Park, R. E.: The City. In *Human Communities.* New York: The Free Press, 1963.

10. Rabkin, R.: Conversion Hysteria as Social Maladaptation. *Psychiatry* 27:349–363, 1964.

11. Rabkin, R., and Rabkin, J.: Delinquency and the Lateral Boundary of the Family. In P. S. Graubard, ed., *Children Against Schools.* Chicago: Follett, 1969, pp. 81–105.

12. Rogers, C. R.: *On Becoming a Person.* Boston: Houghton-Mifflin, 1961.

Chapter Seven: Social Organisms, Networks, and Interfaces:
    Dynamics

1. Sullivan, H. S.: *The Interpersonal Theory of Psychiatry.* New York: Norton, 1953.

2. Perry, H. S.: Commentary. In H. S. Sullivan, *Fusion of Psychiatry and Social Science.* New York: Norton, 1964, pp. 192–198.

3. Sullivan, H. S.: The Illusion of Personal Individuality. *Psychiatry* 13:317–332, 1950.

4. Dewey, J., and Bentley, A.: *Knowing and the Known.* Boston: Beacon Press, 1949.

5. Ryle, G. *The Concept of Mind.* New York: Barnes and Noble, 1949.

6. Hartmann, H.: *Essays on Ego Psychology: Selected Problems in Psychoanalytic Theory.* New York: International Universities Press, 1964.

7. Freud, S.: Analysis of a Case of Hysteria. In *Collected Papers,* vol.

3. London: Hogarth Press, 1953.

8. Holt, R. R.: A Review of some of Freud's Biological Assumptions and their Influence on his Theories. In N. S. Greenfield and W. C. Lewis, *Psychoanalysis and Current Biological Thought*. Madison: University of Wisconsin Press, 1965, pp. 93–124.

9. Freud, S.: *The Problem of Anxiety*. New York: Norton, 1936.

10. Hooper, D., and Roberts, J.: *Disordered Lives: an Interpersonal Account*. New York: Humanities Press, 1968.

11. Sarason, S. B., Levin, M., Goldenberg, I., and Cherlin, D.: *Psychology in Community Settings*. New York: Wiley, 1966.

12. Rausch, H., Goodrich, W. D., and Campbell, J.: Adaptation to the First Years of Marriage. *Psychiatry* 26:368–380, 1963.

13. Freud, S.: From the History of an Infantile Neurosis. In *Collected Papers*, vol. 3. London: Hogarth Press, 1953.

14. Wortis, J.: *Fragments of an Analysis with Freud*. New York: Simon and Schuster, 1954.

15. Bloom, B. L.: The "Medical Model," Miasma Theory and Community Mental Health. *Comm. Ment. Health J.* 1:333–338, 1965.

16. Sussman, M. B.: *Sourcebook in Marriage and the Family*, 3rd ed. Boston: Houghton Mifflin Co., 1968.

17. American Psychiatric Association: *Diagnostic and Statistical Manual: Mental Disorders*. Washington, D.C.: American Psychiatric Association, 1952.

18. Szasz, T.: *The Myth of Mental Illness*. New York: Hoeber, 1961.

19. Menninger, K.: *The Vital Balance*. New York: Viking, 1963.

20. Gruenberg, E. M.: The Social Breakdown Syndrome: Some Origins. *Amer. J. Psychiat.* 123:1481–1489, 1967.

21. Bott, E.: *Family and Social Network*. London: Tavistock, 1957.

22. Speck, R. V.: Personal communication.

23. Southwick, C. H., Beg, M. A., and Siddiqi, M.: Rhesus Monkeys in North India. In I. DeVore, ed., *Primate Behavior*. New York: Holt, Rinehart and Winston, 1965, pp. 111–159.

24. Caplan, G.: Epilogue. In *Concepts of Community Psychiatry: A Framework for Training*. Washington, D.C.: United States Department of Health, Education and Welfare, 1966.

25. Arnold, C. B.: Culture Shock and a Peace Corps Field Mental Health Program. *Comm. Ment. Health J.* 3:53–60, 1967.

26. Oberg, K.: *Consultation in the Brazil-United States Cooperative Health Program, 1942–1955.* Rio de Janeiro: Institute of Inter-American Affairs, 1955.

27. Rabkin, R.: Uncoordinated Communication Between Marriage Partners. *Fam. Process* 6:10–15, 1967.

28. Minuchin, S., Montalvo, B., Guerney Jr., B., Rosman, B., and Schumer, F.: *Families of the Slums.* New York: Basic Books, 1967.

29. Block, D., and Rosenthal, R. A.: Psycho-Social Replication. Paper read at First International Congress of Social Psychiatry, London, August 1964.

30. Meier, R.: Hybrid Vigor in Acculturation: the Puerto Rican Transformation. *Gen. Systems* 6:107–124, 1961.

31. Linton, R.: Marquesan Culture. In A. Kardiner, *The Individual and his Society.* New York: Columbia University Press, 1939, pp. 137–196.

32. *Time Magazine,* November 1, 1967, p. 17.

33. Mattick, I.: Adaptation of Nursery School Techniques to Deprived Children, *J. Amer. Acad. Child Psychiat.* 4:670–700, 1965.

34. Jackson, D. D.: The Individual and the Larger Contexts. *Fam. Process* 6:139–147, 1967.

35. Thompson, C.: Personal communication.

36. Speck, R. V.: Psychotherapy of the Social Network of a Schizophrenic Family. *Fam. Process* 6:208–211, 1967.

37. Menninger, K. *Theory of Psychoanalytic Therapy.* New York: Basic Books, 1958.

Chapter Eight. The Healing Fictions: Pathogenesis

1. Osler, W.: Medicine in the Nineteenth Century. In *Aequanimatas,* Philadelphia: P. Blakeston, 1905.

2. Shapiro, A. K.: A Contribution to a History of the Placebo Effect. *Behav. Sci.* 5:109–135, 1960.

3. Dubois, E. F.: Cornell Conference on Therapy. *N.Y. State J. Med.* 46:1718, 1946.

4. Holmes, O. W.: *Medical Essays, 1842–1882.* Cambridge, Mass.: Riverside Press, 1891.

5. Van Dyke, H. B.: The Weapons of Panacea. *Sci. Monthly* 64:322, 1947.

6. Miner, H.: Body Ritual Among the Nacirema. *Amer. Anthropol.* 58: 503–507, 1956.

7. Butler, S.: *Erewhon, or Over the Range.* New York: Signet Classics, 1960.

8. Rabkin, R.: Conversion Hysteria as Social Maladaptation. *Psychiatry* 27:349–363, 1964.

9. Cummings, E.: *Systems of Social Regulation.* New York: Atherton, 1968.

10. Balint, M.: *The Doctor, His Patient, and the Illness.* New York: International Universities Press, 1957.

11. Weinstein, A.: The Illness Process: Psychosocial Hazards of Disability Programs. *JAMA* 204:209–213, 1968.

12. Richardson, J. G.: *Medicology or Home Encyclopedia of Health.* New York: University Medical Society, 1901.

13. Gurin, G., Veroff, J., and Feld, S.: *Americans View their Mental Health.* New York: Basic Books, 1960.

14. Quoted in *Time,* October 4, 1968, p. 27.

15. Auerswald, E. H.: Interdisciplinary vs. Ecological Approach. *Fam. Process* 7:202–215, 1968.

16. Waddington, C. H.: *The Strategy of the Genes.* London: George Allen and Unwin, 1957.

Chapter Nine. Open Systems: The Theory of Treatment

1. Freud, S.: *New Introductory Lectures on Psycho-Analysis.* New York: Norton, 1933.

2. Glaser, B. G., and Strauss, A. L.: *Awareness of Dying.* Chicago: Aldine, 1965.

3. Bellak, L., and Snell, L.: *Emergency Psychotherapy and Brief Psychotherapy.* New York: Grune and Stratton, 1965.

4. Einstein, A., and Infeld, L.: *The Evolution of Physics.* New York: Simon and Schuster, 1961.

5. Breuer, J., and Freud, S.: *Studies on Hysteria.* New York: Basic Books, 1957.

6. Searles, H.: Oedipal Love in the Countertransference. *Internat. J. Psycho-Anal.* 40:1–11, 1959.

7. Russell, B.: *The Autobiography of Bertrand Russell.* Boston: Little, Brown, 1967.

8. Ibsen, H.: *The Wild Duck*. In *Four Major Plays*, trans. R. Fjelde. New York: Signet Classics, 1965.

9. Ostrovsky, E.: The Anatomy of Cruelty: Antonin Artaud; Louis-Ferdinand Celine. *Arts and Sciences* (NYU) 2:10–13, Spring 1967.

10. Freud, S.: Recommendations for Physicians on the Psycho-Analytic Method of Treatment. In *Collected Papers*, vol. 2. London: Hogarth Press, 1953, pp. 323–333.

11. Strauss, A., ed.: *The Social Psychology of George Herbert Mead*. Chicago: University of Chicago Press, 1956.

12. Marx, K.: Preface to a Contribution to a Critique of Political Economy. In K. Marx and F. Engels, *Selected Works*, vol. 1. Moscow: Foreign Languages Publishing House, 1955.

13. Freud, S.: Analysis of a Case of Hysteria. In *Collected Papers*, vol. 3. London: Hogarth Press, 1953, pp. 13–148.

14. Scheflen, A. E.: Personal communication.

15. Rieff, P.: *Freud: The Mind of the Moralist*. New York: Viking, 1959.

16. Ryle, G.: *The Concept of Mind*. New York: Barnes and Noble, 1949.

Index

Adamov, A., 185
Adler, Alfred, 18
Affect(s), 60–61
 as action or disposition to action, 64, 67
 as aspects of social processes, 62–63, 67, 75
 as defeasible concepts, 66–67
  relevance to psychotherapy of, 67–71
 labeling of, 64–67
 relationship to behavior, 71–73, 75
 performatory nature of, 65–66, 67
 physiological changes and, 63–64
 relativity of, 73
 as representative of substance, Freud's treatment of, 62–63
 repression of, 191–92
 the therapist and system suction, 73–74, 150
American Orthopsychiatric Association, 26
American Psychiatric Association Diagnostic Manuals, 142
American Psychoanalytic Association, 30
Anacreon, 46
Archilochus, 46, 47
Aries, P., 100
Armed Services, 159
Arnold, C. B., 150
Ascriptions, 65–66
Auerswald, E. H., 175

Babel syndrome, 18
Balint, M., 167, 168
Barber, J. X., 63
Bateson, G., 65
Beach, F. A., 105
Beckett, Samuel, 185
Bedford, E., 64
Beers, Clifford, 31
Behavior, ecological approach to, 124–27
 embryology of, and concept of psychic energy, 118–20
 and labeling of affects, 71–73
 instinctive, 119
 physiological model of, 120–21
 and psychotherapy, 127–28
 roulette description of, 120–21
 see also Behaviorism
Behaviorism, modern, Chappell's four points concerning, 50–51, 55–56
 differentiated from behavior therapies, 52
 one-stage conception of behavior, 58–59
 political and moral consequences of, 59
 release as concept of, 55
 Watsonian, 48, 49
Bell, N. W., 34
Bentley, Arthur, 133–34, 135
Bettelheim, Bruno, 87–88
Binet, Alfred, 25–26
Block, D. A., 68, 150–51
Bloom, B. L., 140

Bockhoven, J. S., 31
Bois-Reymond, E. du, 113–14
Bott, E., 144
Brenman, M., 38
Bridgeman, P., 93
British linguistic philosophy, 49
Bronze Age, 22, 23, 45, 48, 96, 97
Buber, Martin, 99
Butler, Samuel, 163–64

Campbell, I., 137
Camus, Albert, 87, 103
Candor, *see* Communications theory
Cards of Identity, 109
Centuries of Childhood, 100
Chappell, V. C., 51, 55
Charles II, 163
Chemotherapy, 30
Chicago Juvenile Court Clinic, 24–26
Child guidance centers, early diag-
    nostic method, 26–27
  juvenile delinquency and, 24–25,
    26
  origin of, 24–26
  proliferation of, 26
  psychoanalytic orientation in, 27–
    28, 30
  effect on orthopsychiatric team, 28,
    31
Cocteau, Jean, 185
Collected Papers (Peirce), 77n
Commission on the Year 2000, 34
Committee on the Next Thirty
    Years, 34
Commonwealth Fund, 26
Communications theory, awareness
    contexts, 189–90, 191–92
  mutual pretense, 181, 184–86,
    192–93
  open communication, 181, 183
  secrets, 181, 182–83, 186, 190–91
  suspected awareness, 181, 182,
    189, 191–92
  blocked communications, 180–81,
    182
  candor, 180, 182–87
  open communications, 181, 183
  significant communications, 181,
    188–89
Cooley, Charles H., 32

Darwin, Charles, 93
Defeasible concept, 66–67
Dennis, Nigel, 109

Depth, *see* Psychoanalysis
Descartes, René, 77, 81, 82–83, 89–
    90
Dewey, John, 19, 32, 59, 65, 83n,
    117, 133–34, 135, 193
Dianetics, 57
Dispositions, 51, 55
Dix, Dorothea, 31
Dr. Zhivago, 48
Double-bind hypothesis, 65
Draper, Theodore, 99
Dream interpretation, 79–80
Driesch, Hans, 114–15
Dubois, E. F., 162
Dynamics, 38
  cycles, 68–69, 99, 100
  spirals, 69, 100
  see also Greece, ancient; Inner
    space; Mass nouns; Structure

Ecology, 114, 118, 121
  classification, 125, 126
  great chain of life, 126–27
  and human behavior, 125–26
  and the illness process, 174–76
  and psychotherapy, 127–30
  and social ideologies, 122–24
  social theory and, 124–25
  succession, process of, 125
Education, and psychotherapy, 86–
    89, 90
Ego, *see* Freud, Sigmund; Psychoan-
    alysis; Unconscious
Einstein, Albert, 77, 182
Electricity, 60, 61–62
Emerson, Ralph Waldo, 32
Emotions, *see* Affect(s)
Energy, psychic, 127
  Freud's concept of, 113–14, 115
  and embryology of behavior, 118–
    20
  and imponderables, 113, 115
  and preformism, 113 114–15
  scientific untenability of, 115–16,
    117–18
  teleological character of, 114
  see also Physiology
Entelechy, 115
Environment, average expectable,
    134, 137–38, 140
  ecological view of, 125–26
Epigenetics, 80, 94
  defined, 104–6

differentiated from preformism, 108–9
Freudian genetic formulations and, 106–8
the social landscape, 176–78, 179
time models and, 107, 108
present *v.* historical perspective, 109–12
Erewhon, 163–64
Erikson, E., 80, 104–5
Euclid, 77

Fallibility, doctrine of, 77, 78, 90
argument for, hallucinations and dreams, 81–83, 90
and therapy, 84–86
Fleiss, W., 38
Foulkes, D., 79–80
Freud, Sigmund, 16*n*, 18, 29–30, 62, 83, 109, 117, 137, 140, 166, 168, 190–91, 193
on behavior and environment, 138–39
concept of psychic energy, 113–14, 115
concept of the unconscious, 47–48, 57, 78–80, 81, 83, 89, 90, 104, 107–8
on fate, 98–99
genetic formulations of, 94, 104–5, 106–8
and metapsychology, 38, 40, 41
neurological theory, question of, 135
reception of ideas of, 182–83
on role of the analyst, 185
time models used by, 101–2
see also Psychoanalysis; Unconscious
Fromm, E., 99
Future-planning, 34–35
Futurists, the, 34

Game theory, 120–21
General Introduction, 79
Genet, Jean, 185
Genetics, 95, 99
Freudian formulations, 94, 104–5, 106–8
preformistic, 93–94
Gide, André 185
Gill, M. M., 38, 40, 41, 106–7
Ginsberg, A., 118–19
Gioscia, V., 102

Glaser, B. G., 190
Goffman E., 67
Goodrich, W. D., 137
Great Britain, 48, 49, 50
Greece, ancient, 21, 23, 43
concept of the community, 45–46, 58
concept of the individual, 45, 58–59
concept of an inner life, 46–47, 58
concept of time, 95–98, 101
human behavior and the *Iliad*, 42
Gruenberg, E. M., 143

Hallucinations, 81–83, 90
Hartmann, H., 134, 138
Hawthorne, Nathaniel, 82
Healy, William, 24–26, 27, 31, 33, 68
Heat, 60
caloric as substance of, 61, 62
mechanical concept of, 61
Henry, Jules, 89
Heraclitus, 37
Hippocrates, 162
Holmes, Oliver Wendell, 60, 61, 62, 162
Holt, R. R., 78–79, 117, 119, 135
Homer, 37, 96
House of Seven Gables, The, 82

Ibsen, Henrik, 185
Iliad, 42–43, 46, 58, 96, 98
Imponderables, 60–64, 120, 127, 187
and psychic energy, 113, 115, 120
see also Affect(s); Electricity; Heat
Innateness, 119
Inner space, 95, 98, 109, 113, 127–28, 186
American criticism of, 50–51
and concept of a release, 55
Early Greek concept of, 46–47, 48, 58–59
outer space as alternative to, 50–51
question of remembering, 56
Soviet criticism of, 48–49
therapy without concept of, 52–58
see also Unconscious
Interfaces, *see* Structure
Interpretation of Dreams, The, 135
Introjection, 186
Iron Age, 21, 22, 23, 98

James, William, 32, 71, 72
Jenkins, R., 27
Joint Commission on Mental Health and Illness, 33
Jones, E., 38
Jones, Richard, 80, 104
Jung, C. G., 169
Juvenile delinquency, 24–25, 26
Juvenile Protective Association, 25

Kamisar, Prof. Yale, 171
Kazin, A., 84, 90
Kennedy, John F., 19
Klemperer, W. A., 148
Knowing and the Known, 133
Knowledge, intuitive, 77–78, 89–90
    relationship to linguistic patterns, 81
Kopkind, A., 35–36

Lamarck, Jean Baptiste, 93
Lange, Carl George, 71, 72
Language, binomial formula, 43–44, 45, 53, 61, 69, 119
    defining process and structure, 94–95, 100–1, 102
    and instinctual-noninstinctual dichotomy, 118–19
    mass nouns, 45
    defined, 43–44
    and early Greek thought, 45–46, 47
    see also Inner Space
Lasswell, H., 35
Lennard, H. L., 69–71
Leontiev, A. N., 48
Linton, R., 152
Logical positivism, 49
Love, romantic, 105n
    see also Affect(s)
Luria, A. R., 48

McLuhan, Marshall, 22–23
Mailer, Norman, 30, 103
Marx, Karl, 189, 193
Mattick, I., 154
Maxwell, J. C. 62, 75
Mead, G. H., 32, 50, 51, 65, 73, 111, 181, 188–89, 190
Meaning, Mead's concept of, 65
Mechanism, *see* Energy, psychic, 119
Medicine, bureacratic *v.* socialistic, 159, 161
    ecology and the illness process, 174–76

government intervention in, 58–59
ideology and society, 159–61, 167
placebos, 161–63, 166, 169–70
social control and regulation, 170–72, 178–79
specialization *v.* general practice, 172–73
transactions between doctor and patient, 163–69
trend toward public health model, 172–74; *see also* Mental health movement
Meditationes de Prima Philosophia, 77n
Meier, R., 152, 153, 154
Menninger, Karl, 26, 143
Meno, 77n, 84
Mental health movement, criticism of development of, 33
    early development of, 31–32
    government intervention in, 35–36
    revolution within, 16–17
    see also Medicine; Social Psychiatry
Metachronicity, 101–4
Metapsychology, 101, 120, 135
    adaptive model, 38, 40–41
    models of and major psychiatric schools, 38–41
Mills, C. Wright, 50
Miner, H., 163
Moral psychiatry, *see* Social psychiatry

National Committee for Mental Hygiene, 26
Natural groups, *see* Communications theory
Networks, *see* Structure, 132
Neurological psychiatry, 16, 17, 18, 19, 37
    and metapsychological models, 38, 39, 40
    and question of the individual psyche, 134–35
Newton, Sir Isaac, 116–17, 182
Nietzsche, Friedrich, 83–84
Nisus formativus, 104

Oberg, K., 149
Oedipus complex, 28, 109, 110, 138, 182–83

Onians, R. B., 96–97
Open systems, *see* Communications theory
Organic theory, 79, 82–83, 85–86, 90
Orthopsychiatric team, 24, 26–27
impact of psychoanalytic theory on, 28, 29, 31
opposition to social psychiatry, 33–34
Orthopsychiatry, *see* Child guidance centers; Orthopsychiatric team
Osler, Sir William, 161
Ostow, M., 115
Outer space, 55, 58, 59
as alternative to inner space, 50–51
see also Behaviorism, modern

Paracelsus, 162
Paramechanical notions, 52–53
Park, Robert E., 125
Participant observer, concept of, 65
Pasternak, Boris, 48
Pathogenesis, 39, 175
see also Medicine
Pavlov, Ivan, 48–49
Peirce, Charles Sanders, 32, 77, 81, 87, 90
see also Fallibility, doctrine of
Performatory statement, 65–66, 67
Perry, H. S., 133
Physiology, as basis of behavior, 120–21
and psychotherapy, 127–28
social theory and, 120, 121–25, 126
see also Energy, psychic
Piaget, Jean, 49
Pinel, P., 16n, 32
Pirie, N. W., 36
Placebos, 161–63, 166, 169–70
Plato, 35, 77, 84, 121–24, 130
Popper, K. R. 83, 85, 89
Preformism, 93–94, 120, 127
and epigenetics, 107, 108–9
Freud's concept of, 113–14, 115
Project for a Scientific Psychology, 113
Psychiatry, defined, 15n
ideological incompatibility within, 18–19
Kraepelinian, 25
psychotherapy and social change, implications of, 34–36

schools of and metapsychology, 38–41
and scientific method, 116–18
two major branches of, 24
see also Mental health movement; Social psychiatry; Structure
Psychoanalysis, 15–16, 17, 18–19, 48, 155
average expectable environment, 134, 137—38, 140
and child guidance centers, 27–28, 30, 31
concept of error in, 83–84
concept of depth (metapsychology), 36–38, 40, 41
decline in popularity of, 29–30
defined, 15n
and epigenetics, 108–9
error of ego psychology, 186
insight, 180, 182–83, 194, 195
and paramechanical notions, 52–53
pessimism of, 193–94
popularity after World War II, 32
professional disenchantment with, 29–30
and question of the unconscious, 79–80
repression, 191–92
therapy, 180, 181–82
see also Freud, Sigmund; Social psychiatry; Unconscious
Psychology, early American, 25–26
Psychosocial replication, 68

Rapaport, David, 18, 38, 40, 41, 106–7
Rausch, H., 137
Release(s), 43, 74, 193
as behavioristic concept, 55–56
and concept of inner space, 55
defined, case histories illustrating, 52–58
Republic, 121–24, 130
Revisionism, 18
Rieff, P., 47–48, 193
Rumford, B. T., 61
Russell, Bertrand, 184
Ryle, Gilbert, 19, 50, 52, 64, 134, 135, 194

Sanford, R. N., 86
Sapir, E., 102

Sappho, 46
Sarason, S. B., 137
Scheflen, A. E., 191
Schneirla, T. C., 119
Scientific method, and question of psychic energy, 115–16, 117–18
Snell, B., 37, 45
Snuggling, 149–50, 156
Social organisms structures, see Structure
Social psychiatry, 37, 118
   attempt to integrate into psychoanalytic theory, 18–20
   challenge to traditional psychiatry, 23–24
   and concept of inner space, refutation of vulgar behaviorism, 50–53
   and contemporary social problems, 20–21
   defined, 15n
   development of, 32
   emergence of as major contemporary psychiatric frontier, 33–34
   epigenetics and, 108–12, 176–78, 179
   and future-planning question, 34–35
   as independent science, theoretical question, 15–20, 23–24
   initial adoption of, 17
   language and, defining the intangible, 94–95
   and mental health movement revolution, 16–17
   and metapsychological models, 38–41
   nexus of pathology in, 183
   in the 19th century, effect of Civil War on, 31–32
   success of in New England, 31, 32
   and orthopsychiatry, 26
   pessimism or optimism question, 193–94
   political implications of use of, 35–36
   and present trend toward community medicine, 172–74
   question of process and structure, 92–93
   question of remembering, 56–58
   relation to psychoanalysis, 181–83

therapy in absence of theoretical groundwork, 181
   and concepts of inner space, 52–58
   question of education, 86–89, 90, 181
   self-knowledge v. social competence, 181, 194–95
   see also Behaviorism, modern; Communications theory; concepts of throughout index
Social sciences, new developments in and future-planning, 34–35
Society, problems of radical solutions, 20–23
   see also Social psychiatry
Socrates, see Plato
Southwick, C. H., 146
Soviet Union, 48–49, 50
Speck, R. V., 155
Sraffa, Piero, 49
Stranger, The, 103
Strauss, A., 190
Structure, 92–93, 94–95, 107, 108, 120
   adaptive point of view, the psychotherapist and the environment, 137–40
   individual and environment, 131–32
   interfaces/interface dynamics, 132, 146–47, 156, 191
      accentuation, 151–52
      assimilation, 153
      communalization, 153
      conflict, 153
      defined, 147–48
      dissolution, 152
      and the group, 152–56
      induction, 150
      penetration, 149–50, 156–57
      resonance, 150–51
      selective combination, 153
      shock, 148–49, 150
      stationing, 151
      treatment strategies, 155–57
   networks, 132
      classification of, 144
      defined, 143–45
      interfaces and, 146–47
      redefinition of personality through, 145–46
   organismic approach, criticism of, 141–43

personal individuality question,
132–35
variability of environment, 134,
135–37
Sullivan, Harry Stack, 18, 20, 32, 50,
59, 65, 84–85, 132–33, 135, 145,
189–90
Sussman, H. B., 142
Sydenham, Thomas, 162
Szasz, T., 67, 143

Thomas, W. I., 32
Thompson, Clara, 155
Thoreau, Henry David, 32
Thrasymachus' argument, 121–24
Time, cyclical, 100–1, 103–4, 108,
111–12
as a fixed pattern, 100, 103
four views of in psychotherapy,
98–101
historical, 98, 102, 109–11
linear, 99, 102
as a point, 99–100, 102–3
as preformed fate, 95–98, 101, 102
Topography, see Fallibility, doctrine
of: Unconscious

Unconscious, 40, 41, 57, 76–77, 81,
83, 104, 107–8, 109, 120, 127,
191
and classical Greek tradition, 78–
79
and concept of inner space, 47–48
and concept of psychic energy,
113, 114, 120
resistance, 83–84, 85–86, 89, 90
question of education, 86
timelessness of, 99
United States, 48, 50

Veterans Administration, 33, 159
Vico, Giambattista, 15, 20, 21
Vitalism, 114–15, 117, 118, 119, 127
Vygotsky, L. S., 49, 87, 88

Watson, John B., 50, 51
Waddington, C. H., 176
Watts, Alan, 100
Weinstein, A., 168
White, William Alanson, 32, 50
Whorf, B. L., 44, 61, 69, 94, 95
Wild Duck, The, 185
Wittgenstein, Ludwig, 49, 50
Wortis, Joseph, 139